Winter Blues Survival Guide

Feb 2014

Also from Norman E. Rosenthal

WINTER BLUES:
Everything You Need to Beat Seasonal Affective Disorder,
Fourth Edition

For more information,
visit the author's website: *http://normanrosenthal.com*

Winter Blues Survival Guide

A Workbook for Overcoming SAD

Norman E. Rosenthal

Christine M. Benton

THE GUILFORD PRESS
New York   London

© 2014 The Guilford Press
A Division of Guilford Publications, Inc.
72 Spring Street, New York, NY 10012
www.guilford.com

Printed in the United States of America

This book is printed on acid-free paper.

Last digit is print number: 9   8   7   6   5   4   3   2   1

Library of Congress Cataloging-in-Publication Data

Rosenthal, Norman E., author.
    Winter blues survival guide : a workbook for overcoming SAD /
  Norman E. Rosenthal and Christine M. Benton.
        pages   cm
    Includes bibliographical references and index.
    ISBN 978-1-4625-1232-4 (pbk.)
    1. Seasonal affective disorder.   2. Depression, Mental.   3. Affective
disorders.   4. Self-care, Health.   I. Benton, Christine M., author.
II. Title.
    RC545.R673 2014
    616.85'27—dc23
                                                                2013020201

Contents

Purchasers may download and print select practical tools from this book at *www.guilford.com/rosenthal3-forms*.

Acknowledgments

We would like to thank our editor at The Guilford Press, Kitty Moore, for her encouragement and infectious enthusiasm during the writing of this workbook. Thanks also to research assistants Dan McQuaid and Shebna Garcon for their help throughout the writing process. Finally, we are mutually grateful for a fruitful collaboration and hope this workbook helps all those who have been struggling with SAD symptoms lead happier, more fulfilling lives.

Winter Blues Survival Guide

Introduction

☐ Do fall leaves and the first chilly days make you want to crawl under a quilt and stay there until spring?

☐ While your friends are joking about having put on a few pounds thanks to holiday sweets, are you buying larger clothes in February—along with bags of chips and cookies you barely glance at in summer?

☐ Do you tend to feel down, irritable, and tired during winter, a state that's hard to picture when the joy of summer returns?

☐ Do projects you started in August slow to a halt if you haven't finished them by October?

☐ Do romance and sex migrate from the top of your to-do list during the warm months to the bottom by winter?

Nodding your head with familiarity at any or all of the above means you may be one of the millions of people in the world who suffer from seasonal affective disorder (SAD), a pattern of depression that comes and goes in synch with the yearly cycle of shifting daylight and changing temperatures. It means you probably know very well how difficult it is to have your mood, mental focus, energy, and sense of well-being plummet when the days get short. If you answered "yes" to all five of the preceding questions, you may be facing a truly SAD situation. Perhaps you feel as if every year you are robbed of months of productivity and contentment. Instead of getting ahead at work, relishing the company of family and friends, pursuing the leisure activities that give life its luster, your life seems to enter a fog as you struggle to get out of bed every day. Seasonal affective disorder, or SAD, varies in severity

1

like any other condition, but even in its milder forms it can deny you the full enjoyment of your life and leave you wondering whether you'd be better off bedding down with the bears until the crocuses appear.

It doesn't have to be this way. With the help of this book, you can reclaim the light—and your life—during all four seasons, from spring's bright promise to summer's abundance, through autumn's vibrant palette, all the way to December's darkest days. The most common form of SAD is the *winter* blues, but for some people seasonal depression makes the intense sun of summer feel like an unrelenting antagonist. They get the *summertime* blues. Whatever time of year brings depression for you, there is help in the following chapters. The key is to understand how SAD operates, and particularly how it affects you uniquely, so that you can prepare for what the seasons have in store for you and possibly prevent the worst of the effects that seasonal depression can deliver.

Think about it for a minute:

What could you gain if you were *aware* of exactly how the seasons affect you?

How could you *prepare* so the change of seasons doesn't hit you so hard?

How much better would your life be if awareness and preparation helped you *prevent* the worst of your symptoms?

This book is your SAD Solution APP:
A for *awareness*, P for *preparation*, P for *prevention*.

Because SAD often arrives predictably at the same time every year for you, you have the opportunity to plan ahead. With this workbook, you can keep track of exactly how your symptoms wax and wane, figure out which preventive measures and treatments will work best for you, and then spend your high-energy months equipping yourself for your low-energy months. Simple checklists, summaries of facts, and handy logs can help organize information about your experience with SAD that is usually lost in the morass of depression. This book can serve as your diary of SAD, an indispensable reference to turn to when you need to recall exactly when you started light therapy and how long it took for the effects to kick in . . . how you got through last year's winter holidays (or the kids' summer vacation) so much more smoothly than the year before . . . what types of meals kept your weight low and your self esteem high . . . which friends made it easy to socialize without pressure . . . how you managed to add pleasure to every day instead of losing most days to agonizing over unfinished tasks . . . and all the other little details about what helps you overcome the effects of SAD—and actually enjoy the winter. Perhaps most important, a workbook can make it easier to sort through your thoughts and your experiences to find the best path to well-being when that task may seem overwhelming.

> ***The take-home message:*** **The change of seasons affects us all, but it doesn't have to make us feel SAD. The goal of this book is to help you stay up and running through the winter— not down and out.**

I am a prime example. As I was studying seasonality at the National Institute of Mental Health (NIMH), gathering reams of data thanks to the insights of many generous patients who were willing to describe their experiences with the changes of season throughout their lives, I realized that I had been suffering from SAD since arriving in New York City for my psychiatric residency. As the sunlight ebbed away, so did my energy and zest. I gritted my teeth and soldiered on through the winter. Cookies and candy became a dependable—although short-lived— source of comfort, but I paid the price for this indulgence, as indicated by the needle on my bathroom scale. When spring came, everything just seemed to get better.

You may be able to go from severe SAD one winter to mild winter blues the next and finally to no symptoms at all if you attack seasonality from a number of angles.

The biblical proverb "Physician, heal thyself" took on a new meaning for me, and as my colleagues and I amassed information on remedies for SAD I realized how valuable it would be—not just to me personally but to all who could benefit from our research—for me to follow my own advice. And so I did. I started using a light box, and to this day I seldom travel without one during the winter. I repainted the walls in my home a bright white and pruned trees that were blocking the sun from pouring through my windows. To reduce stress, I began to exercise regularly, and I learned transcendental meditation (and became so impressed with the results that I wrote a book about it). And I learned all I could about carbohydrate cravings and changed my diet to emphasize lean protein, vegetables, and low-impact carbs and to minimize the high-impact carbs: pure sugars and white starches. Perhaps most important, as I was learning through experimentation what treatments, environmental modifications, and lifestyle changes work for me, I taught myself to accept the limitations that still bothered me on some winter days, allowing myself to get done whatever I could. I made it a point to attend social events even when I didn't feel like it ahead of time and usually ended up surprised by how the company of others lifted my spirits. Although I accept that winter may not feel as good as summer, I have reclaimed a sense of well-being by reversing the low moods of winter. Even in winter I have maintained my weight at its summer level, and I have regained the ability to do almost as much work in February as in July. I have beaten SAD (most of the time). I no longer qualify for a diagnosis of the dis-

> *In one recent large study the average person with SAD had endured 14 winter depressions before entering the program being studied—and half had never been treated for any of the symptoms. How long can you wait before getting the help you deserve?*

order, nor do I feel the milder effects of the winter blues (except for brief spells). By following my own advice, I feel like I can live fully all year long. Now I'd like to help you do so too.

My involvement in SAD research put me on a straight path to resolving seasonal symptoms. Most people aren't so lucky. Many people remain undiagnosed—and untreated—even when they present their doctors with a history that matches the diagnostic criteria for a variety of reasons:

- Light therapy, despite its proven effectiveness, seems "alternative" to some clinicians.

- Some people don't talk about their symptoms because they believe what they're experiencing isn't real. (If everyone feels somewhat down during winter, it couldn't be true depression, could it?)

- It's easy for depressed people to feel like SAD is "my own fault" rather than a problem that can be solved readily.

- Finally, it is not always intuitive to think in terms of the seasons. We may blame our low mood on something bad that happened at the end of last summer—rather than seeing it as part of a cycle.

It has taken astute awareness by thousands of individuals to help us get a clear picture of SAD, and it is often individuals with seasonal depression who have helped educate others and put them on the path to feeling better year-round. Bridget, a woman I introduced first in *Winter Blues,* is a great example of the power of self-awareness. Bridget said that she had always disliked winter, but that it was only as a young adult that she began to experience a pattern of seasonal symptoms. And it was only in her mid-30s, when she came to our program in Washington, D.C., that she could fit the puzzle pieces together so well that her SAD appeared in sharp relief. The biggest problem for Bridget may have been that, as she said, for years she was like the grasshopper, singing and playing all summer and not worrying about the winter. It was only when the leaves began to turn color and the autumn catalogs arrived, and by connecting her experiences to what was going on around her, that she was able to get a handle on SAD. By observing and reviewing her experiences closely, Bridget learned when her first symptoms began, when they peaked, and when they started to subside. She noticed that her SAD took the form of extreme fatigue, carb cravings, depressed feelings, and irritability. She also realized that when she went to the Caribbean for a winter vacation two years in a row, she felt better shortly after arriving and then bad again almost the minute she returned to the cold North. By reviewing how her symptoms had manifested in the different places she had lived over the years, she noticed that the farther north she resided, the earlier in the fall her depression began and the later in the spring it ended. Pairing that observation with the fact that she hated her dimly lit office and made frequent visits to the bright photocopying room, she hit on the main trigger for her SAD syndrome: light. Light was so central to her seasonal experiences that she was eager to try light therapy and thrilled to find that it worked well for her all by itself.

Other patients of mine have had similar experiences: the more they accurately understood the influence of the seasons on their mood, mind, and physical well-being, the more they were able to zero in on the remedies and treatments that would counteract their symptoms. Like Bridget and thousands of others, you can determine what makes you SAD and use the power of that understanding to prepare and ultimately prevent the seasons from beating you down. Your SAD Solution APP is yours for the taking in Part I of this book.

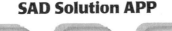

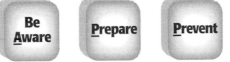

In Part II you'll find out how to identify and apply a wide selection of treatments for those symptoms that still affect you annually, as well as ongoing help with awareness, preparation, and prevention that can help you make the most of each remedy or strategy:

SAD Solution APP-T

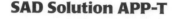
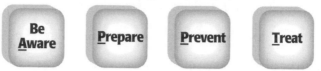

To get you off on the right foot, what brought you to this book? What would you like to get out of it?

☐ 1. I'm tired of feeling so down in winter and don't want to put up with it any longer. There must be a better way.

☐ 2. I know I have SAD and have gotten a lot out of using a light box but still don't feel as good as I'd like to once the days get shorter. I want to do better.

☐ 3. I have a family member who sinks into depression every fall but denies there's anything really wrong or anything that can be done about it. I want to help.

☐ 4. I have read *Winter Blues* but am attracted to the hands-on approach offered by a workbook.

★ KEY POINTS

If you're in group 1 . . .

You can make great use of this whole book. Work through it from front to back (or cherry-pick the sections that seem most relevant to *you*), becoming aware in detail of how the seasons affect you, learning about your treatment options (both with professional help and via self-help), and then picking the course or courses of action that seem best and easiest for you. If you haven't yet learned much about SAD, consider reading the fourth edition of *Winter Blues* (2013) for comprehensive, up-to-date scientific advice and information—or just have it on hand to refer to when you need more on a particular SAD subject.

If you're in group 2 . . .

You'll probably be able to sail through Part I of this book, although using the tools we offer to take a close look at your own SAD experience may reveal important information that you can use to get the most out of Part II. Choose the remedies and treatments that appeal to you and you stand an excellent chance of bumping up the positive effects you're already getting from your light therapy and greeting the colder days with equanimity, or even positive anticipation of the distinct pleasures of winter.

If you're in group 3 . . .

Pass this book along. For those who are convinced they don't have a "real" problem or that even if they do there's no help for it, the first few chapters offer a compendium of facts about SAD—who has it, how it varies, and how it differs from normal reactions to the changes in season—that can be a revelation to doubters. For your own information—and your relative's—*Winter Blues* might be a valuable resource too, especially the chapter that offers advice for family and friends.

If you're in group 4 . . .

That's a major reason we wrote this book: to give you the practical information you need in the easiest and most accessible form.

*   *   *

The power you'll gain in this book is the power to choose: With the information and tools in the following pages you'll gain the flexibility to make choices about how to conduct your life so that you can live it to the fullest, without restrictions by the seasons. Let there be light!

Part I

Everything You Need to Know to Feel Less SAD

What Do You Know about Your Relationship with the Seasons?

What is your favorite season? Rank them in order of preference, 1 for the time of year you like best, 4 for the season you'd most like to erase from the calendar:

_____ Spring

_____ Summer

_____ Autumn

_____ Winter

The goal of this little exercise is not to reveal that you almost surely ranked summer or spring number 1 and winter number 4 (if you have winter SAD) *but to show how easily you made these choices.* You're probably aware on some level that you've been greeting the darker months the way you would a recurring nightmare, and yet it may have taken you years to seek help for SAD. Why? The answer lies in the complicated relationship that human beings have with the seasons and how it has evolved through history. Understanding this rela-

> *A sad tale's best for winter.*
> —WILLIAM SHAKESPEARE,
> *A Winter's Tale*

tionship is an important first step in developing the awareness you need to make *your* relationship with the seasons an amicable one.

Be Aware

HOW AWARE ARE YOU OF THE SEASONS' EFFECTS?

This book is all about increasing your awareness so you can beat SAD. If you are just starting to look at the possibility that you have some version of seasonality, you may have gone for years without fully recognizing your symptoms and their impact on your life. If you are already addressing your seasonality but think you could feel even better, there's probably more you can discover about your relationship with the seasons to gain additional improvements.

Our senses tell us when the seasons are changing—we feel the temperature dropping or rising, we smell flowers blooming or fallen leaves decaying, we're greeted by varying degrees of sunlight when we open our eyes to the new day. The calendar confirms what time of year it is. So why delve more deeply? Paying attention to exactly how the current season affects your mood, your energy, your appetite for food or sex, or how well you sleep may have seemed as

> *To be interested in the changing seasons is a happier state of mind than to be hopelessly in love with spring.*
> —GEORGE SANTAYANA,
> The Life of Reason

useful as asking yourself how one breath of air differs from the next—at least until the pang of regret for the end of picnic weather and beach days is replaced by full-blown dread that's hard to shake. Now your relationship with the seasons is more complicated. A number of preconceived notions can keep you from understanding why you may have a love–hate relationship with this aspect of the natural world and from finding a comfortable place in it.

☐ **Have you assumed that you shouldn't "let the seasons get you down" since they don't seem to trouble those around you?**

It's true: Many people can feel generally as happy in winter as in summer, just as upbeat and productive in fall as in spring. If you're surrounded by these people, as you probably have been all your life, you may very well have concluded you should be equally resilient. As a result, you've probably tried to shrug off the fact that for you the changing colors of autumn are accompanied by fear of the cold, cold months to follow. You may have tried to put on a good face at the holidays even though you were in a serious funk and didn't feel like joining the party.

Efforts like these may even have helped to an extent. Maybe you pushed yourself to go to that New Year's Eve party (perhaps because you felt you *ought to)* and ended up feeling much better in the company of friends than if you had hunkered down alone at home. (Socializing when you don't feel like it, *at least sometimes,* is one measure that I advocate.) But if you didn't succeed in acting cheerful during holiday gatherings or in leaving home at all for a party, you may well have blamed yourself. In that case, with your mind caught up in guilt and shame, you could hardly be fully aware of how the seasons were affecting you. And if you persisted in pushing yourself to act like nothing was wrong, denial of the problem also limited your awareness of exactly what was going on between you and the seasons. Sadly, with awareness blocked, so is the understanding that could help you manage or even solve the problem.

☐ **Or do you believe the opposite—that everyone feels the way you do when winter comes, and puts up with it—so you should too?**

One woman I treated had endured SAD for several decades before seeking treatment. When asked why, she said she had assumed everyone felt the same way she did! Many people with varying degrees of SAD believe that everyone deals with winter without complaining, and therefore complaining would be a sign of weakness. As noted above, everyone *doesn't* dislike winter. The people around you aren't all being stoic, some even love winter. And for those who do dislike winter, not everyone puts up with winter difficulties. Many adopt the remedies outlined in this book. (The fact that you aren't talking about your winter problems may be what's keeping you from hearing about how many others have SAD and what they're doing about it!) As to those who do try to grin and bear their winter blues, I respectfully suggest that they would feel better if they beat the winter blues—and so would you.

☐ **Do you believe you're to blame for your winter problems, and therefore you should just keep trying to deny them?**

Most people with SAD *do* feel different, but many believe they *shouldn't* be different. As explained above, some believe everyone has the same problems but puts up with them, and others believe no one has the same problems and therefore they must be imagining them. Both assumptions can lead to self-blame—either you're causing the problems or you're just not "tough enough" to rise above them. Feeling like you are to blame for your SAD symptoms can be a disempowering feeling, leading you to believe that you are not entitled to relief because it is your fault. When you believe you're not entitled to relief, the only solution is to try to pretend the problem doesn't exist. Limiting your awareness in that way can keep you from discovering exactly what you need among the remedies in this book to feel better.

The remedy if you're blaming yourself for SAD is (1) to recognize that it is a biological variant and therefore *not* your fault and (2) to ask yourself "Why not treat it as you would any condition?"

💡 **You may find it difficult to shed the belief that you are somehow to blame for your seasonality. Accepting SAD as a legitimate illness that limits what you can do when depressed can be an ongoing struggle. Even if you recognize the facts above, they are easy to forget, especially when you're feeling down. You may find yourself accepting on some days and resisting on others. Because lack of acceptance can make you feel so much worse and may lead you to deny yourself the help you need, I'll take the liberty of gently reminding you throughout this book that you have a right to get the help you need and to minimize stress so you can cope with SAD.**

☐ **Have you told yourself that fighting the seasons is futile?**

Maybe you've told yourself there was nothing you could do about the seasons' effects on you because summer, fall, winter, and spring are going to keep cycling through the year, taking you along with them. Happily, this assumption is usually wrong. You certainly can't stop the seasons from coming and going. But you *can* prepare for them in ways you haven't done so far. Instead of bracing themselves for the inevitable crash (while hoping against hope that they won't get so depressed this winter), many people anticipate SAD symptoms: They take specific steps. For example, they book winter trips to sunny locales or repaint their living quarters a bright, light color.

Myth Buster: Some people hesitate to seek help for SAD symptoms because they figure if their depression occurs only at certain times of the year it's not "real depression." The fact is that SAD falls under the umbrella of major depression. And that doesn't mean SAD is milder across the board or less significant or worthy of help. SAD can be just as severe as any other type of major depression.

☐ **Do you believe that looking back at the discomfort you've suffered in the past is simply wallowing and self-indulgent?**

There's a distinct difference between reflection and wallowing. Reflection leads to solutions; wallowing does not. At risk of overgeneralizing, it may be no coincidence that the cultures inhabiting the regions of the world where SAD is most prevalent (northern North America and Europe) tend to value independence and self-determination highly. Winter has taught us that it is important to fend for ourselves. But we can take this attitude too far—especially these days, when so much information and help is available. By all means, be independent, but also make use of these resources.

Sarah sank into a deep depression 3 years ago after losing her job in marketing in November. She managed to pull herself out of it in April and started looking for a new job in earnest. She got a position as an assistant curator at a local museum—her dream job. But the new field was a challenge for her, and by fall she was starting to get negative feedback from her boss. At the end of the year she was fired. Sarah had another tough winter but found a new job in March. She also started dating someone that she really liked, and everything was great until October,

> *How much progress is really possible if we ignore the events that hold us back year after year?*

Linear versus Cyclical Time

Ancient civilizations were intimately connected with the cycle of the seasons (as well as the cycle of day and night). Rituals and customs marked the milestones of every year and often incorporated references to the sun and other aspects of the natural world. This focus on the repetition of annual events instilled a cyclical sense of time that kept people tuned in to the seasons and the changes they brought. Then, in more recent centuries, a sense of linear time began to predominate. The Judeo-Christian tradition connected people's behavior with consequences imposed by God—no longer could individuals anticipate starting with a clean slate every year. The succession of dynasties cemented the idea of linear time in China, and other cultures began to view time as an arrow—fleeting, unidirectional, and irretrievable. A sense of linear time certainly promoted the idea of progress, but in the process we have overlooked the importance of cyclical time—as exemplified by the changing seasons.

when she started fighting with her boyfriend and calling in sick at work. Looking back, she describes the winter that year as "gloomy." But it was all forgotten once the summer returned. In the fall, her boyfriend broke up with her, saying she was just too irritable to be around. She went to see her doctor for "exhaustion," and he prescribed a new diet, exercise, and asked her to come back in 6 weeks.

Examined along a straight timeline (remember those datelines you had to draw in social studies class?), Sarah's recurrent problems may seem unconnected. Naturally she got depressed after her job loss and subsequent relationship problems. But if you look at her recent history in a cyclical sense, it's pretty obvious that her depressions and related problems always started in the fall and eased in the spring. Viewed through this more useful lens, her doctor might have considered SAD as a diagnosis right away.

Of course, I am not suggesting that we rid ourselves entirely of our sense of linear time. That perspective does make progress possible—including, ironically, the progress that we've made in insulating ourselves from the effects of the seasons, from the development of air conditioning to the prevalence of artificial light.

Fortunately, in recent years scientists and the general public have renewed their interest in the cycles of our natural world by exploring biological rhythms, and this shift laid the foundation for the discovery of the phenomenon now known as SAD. Throughout this book I'll ask you to do some exploring of your own, taking a new look at the biological rhythms that connect you with the cycle of the seasons and also with the cycle of sunlight and darkness. Understanding how we are all connected to these grander rhythms of the world is the first step in getting acquainted with your own unique form of seasonality. It is a love–hate relationship for anyone suffering the symptoms of SAD, but as with an irritating relative that you can't disown, it's a relationship that you can manage by knowing exactly what you're dealing with.

Be Aware   FIRST STEPS TOWARD AWARENESS: STARTING TO EXPLORE YOUR OWN SAD

To get a glimpse at your own SAD awareness, answer these questions:

When did you first notice a strong preference for one season over another?

☐ Childhood   ☐ Adolescence   ☐ Adulthood

How has that preference evolved over the years?

☐ Weakened   ☐ Intensified   ☐ Varied from year to year   ☐ Stayed about the same

When did these preferences become a problem for you?

_____ Year of age or:

☐ During school years   ☐ In college   ☐ As a working adult   ☐ During parenthood

You may not have been able to answer these deceptively simple questions as quickly as you did the first exercise in this chapter. A habit of ignoring or minimizing seasonal discomfort can make your years with SAD seem like they passed in a blur. One goal of this book is to help you re-create your SAD history because it holds the keys to identifying the best remedies. If your best winters were the four years you spent at the University of New Mexico, you know that having sunshine every day really helps you. If your worst winters were those when you had your first job, where your desk was in a windowless cubicle with low light, you know that even a great job won't be so good for you if it keeps you in the dark all day. If you did better in winter when each of your children was a baby and you took long walks outdoors early in the morning, you know that taking a brisk walk by yourself at that time of day could really boost your mood even in January.

People between their 20s and 40s seem to be most susceptible to SAD, but many diagnosed during that period distinctly remember disliking winter much earlier—they just didn't think it was important to register their changing feelings back then.

How often have you found yourself brushing off the dread that accompanies another approaching winter?

☐ Never   ☐ Seldom   ☐ Occasionally   ☐ Often

How many winters in a row have you told yourself to look forward to better times ahead and stop dwelling on the past?

_____

Choose one significant date in fall or winter—Thanksgiving, Christmas, Hanukkah, your birthday or a family member's or friend's, the start of school, etc.—or in summer if you have summer SAD and write down what you remember about your experience that day over the last 3–5 years. Don't spend a lot of time on this; just quickly jot down your general memory of the day—how you felt, whether you enjoyed yourself, and the like:

Last year: _____

Two years ago: _____

Three years ago: _____

Four years ago: _____

Five years ago: _____

What did you learn from the preceding exercise? If you can't remember much, it might be because, like many people with SAD, you pass fall and winter days in something of a fog. Or it could be because you would prefer to forget those seemingly endless days—understandable, but somewhat counterproductive. This workbook is your chance to call up those memories to make use of them, not to torment yourself.

For those years you were able to record something, did you notice a pattern? Are your memories generally positive, negative, or neutral? Do you associate that date with a specific feeling—blue, down, cross, angry, elated, content? What about your physical state? Tired, energized, comfortable, achy, ill? Do you recall changes in daily sleep length and food intake (more in winter, less in summer)? Observations like these are the jigsaw pieces that will ultimately fit together into a coherent picture of your SAD and will help you solve the puzzle of your seasonality.

LIGHT: CENTER STAGE IN SEASONALITY

Living on planet Earth, we are aware that the sunlight envelops us; it's part of our natural habitat. Everyone else seems to take it for granted. But for those of us who have SAD, the only time we *may* take it for granted is when there is plenty of it (like the grasshopper in Aesop's fable). When it isn't there, we *really* miss it. We may not be fully aware of the emotional, cognitive, and physical effects that seasonal changes in sunlight exert on us, but we know something feels wrong. The effects of these changes in sunlight are at the heart of seasonality.*

---

*Summer SAD is an exception. There the influences of the sun seem to have a deleterious effect.

ⅠＡⅠ SCIENCE

What We Know about the Power of the Light in SAD

The seasons themselves are the result of the changing angle of sunlight on the earth caused by our planet's axial tilt as it makes a revolution around the sun over the year. We have some interesting data to back up the centrality of light in SAD:

- People who are living at the most northerly latitudes, and therefore receive the least daily sunlight in fall and winter, tend to become depressed earlier in the year and start feeling better later than those living farther south. We've seen this in individuals who have lived at different latitudes (Canada and New York versus Washington, D.C.).

- SAD is more common at higher latitudes. See the table below.

- Some people with SAD instinctively gravitate toward brighter artificial light in the winter. My patients have reported feeling better sitting in front of their plant lights at home, going grocery shopping at night, spending a lot of time

Prevalence of SAD and the Winter Blues by Latitude

City/state/country	Latitude	Prevalence (% of sample)		
		SAD	WB	Total
Sarasota, Florida	27°	1.4	2.6	4.0
Maryland	39°	6.3	10.4	16.7
New York City	40°	4.7	12.5	17.2
Nashua, New Hampshire	42°	9.7	11.0	20.7
Fairbanks, Alaska	65°	9.2	19.1	28.3
Stockholm, Sweden	59°	3.9	13.9	17.8
Helsinki, Finland	59°	7.1	11.8	18.9
Oslo, Norway	59°	14.0	12.6	24.6
Reykjavik, Iceland	64°	3.8	7.6	11.3
Tromsö, Norway	69°	13.7	10.7	24.4
Nagoya, Japan	35°	0.9	0.8	1.7

in a bright office photocopying room, and routinely turning on every light in the home during the winter months. But some people don't have this instinctive light hunger and need to teach themselves to gravitate to light.

- People with vision problems that reduce the amount of light that can enter the eye are more vulnerable to SAD. This first came to my attention when a middle-aged man who had SAD and no other risk factors revealed that he had a cataract in one eye.

*   *   *

Looking back, how have you reacted to changes in the amount and intensity of sunlight? (Check off all that apply to you.)

☐ I get sleepy and cranky when I have to get up in the dark, go to work, and come home in the dark.

☐ I feel better taking a walk in the snow on sunny days, even though the sunniest days are often the coldest where I live.

☐ I have no problem with a day or two of rain, but if it lasts for a week, I start to feel down, and it's not because I'm bored—I don't even want to go out.

☐ I don't like "cozy," dimly lit restaurants in winter.

☐ I've changed jobs because my workspace was dark and there's no relief in the rest of the office.

☐ I love the feel of the summer sun on my skin, but when I'm outdoors on the brightest days I try to keep my back to the sun or I start to feel agitated and scattered.

☐ I love to be surrounded by color, but I repainted the room I spend most of my time in white because the darker walls depressed me.

SELF-AWARENESS AS POWER

You're undoubtedly reading this book because you know you've been experiencing a pattern of SAD symptoms to a sufficient degree for long enough that it's become unpleasant at best and sometimes intolerable. You still might be surprised by what you have revealed through the simple exercises you've done so far in this chapter. It is this kind of self-awareness—and some record-keeping that this book makes easy—that gives *you* the power to have nicer holidays, a happier birthday, or a more productive start to the school year.

Knowing the *pattern* of your SAD symptoms is, in fact, one of three keys to gaining power over seasonality. Being aware of the extent of the *variation* of your symptoms from year to year is the second key. The third key is understanding the *impact* of your seasonality: How much does SAD get in your way?

In Chapter 2 you will have the opportunity to self-administer part of the questionnaire used by professionals to assess these three aspects of your seasonality. But to get yourself thinking in an empowering way, review the following questions. You can just let these questions percolate in your mind for now, or go ahead and jot down what comes to mind if you wish:

When during the year do you first notice your mood or energy level starting to sink?

_____

When do symptoms first get the better of you?

_____

What symptom gets to you first?

_____

What happens after that?

☐ Fatigue? ☐ Loss of inter- ☐ Loss of ☐ Sleeping
              est in fun   energy?   problems?
☐ Pessimism? activities?
                          ☐ Changes in ☐ Other?
☐ Sorrow?   appetite?

_____

_____

Do your symptoms come on gradually or hit you over the head all at once?

_____

Do they start at the same time every year or fluctuate (sometimes starting in fall, sometimes at the start of winter)?

_____

Do your symptoms vary in intensity from year to year, with some winters being truly awful and others seeming more tiring than painful?

_____

In the last 5 years, which was your worst winter? _____

Which was your best? _____

Why do you think that was so? _____

Do you feel plain old good in summer or somewhat hyper (getting little sleep, taking on too many tasks, talking too fast or too much)?

_____

Do your symptoms appear when the shortest days occur (near the winter solstice, December 21), or do they start soon after the days start getting shorter (after the summer solstice, June 21) and wane as soon as they start getting longer (in January)?

_____

THE PATTERN OF YOUR SEASONALITY

Everyone's SAD is unique. In broad strokes we can say you either have the winter blues or summer SAD, but within those two general patterns lie a number of variations. One example is the winter *plus* summer pattern where you have seasonal difficulties at both times of year. You may have noted at the beginning of this chapter that winter is the toughest season for you, but is it just winter, or is fall uncomfortable for you as well? You might experience only a month or two of depression—or 6 months. Some people suffer from depression year-round but find that it may get worse at certain predictable times of year. It's important to identify your pattern of seasonality because it can make a big difference in your treatment.

For winter SAD: If you experience winter symptoms for only a couple months, diligently using light therapy during that time may be all you need. If you have depression year-round, but worse in winter, you may want to use light therapy year-round but augment it with antidepressant medication and/or some of the other options discussed in this book during the darkest months. If your depression is fairly severe in winter, you will probably want to use light therapy and anything else that helps bring you back to normal.

For summer SAD or winter-plus-summer SAD: Do you have the opposite problem in summer and find yourself so overenergized that you run from one task to another and are so frazzled that you get little done? Some people become so hyper during the longest days that their sensitivity to the light level makes maximum sun almost as harmful to them as minimal sun is to someone with the winter blues or with a summer–winter pattern. In that case occasionally pulling the blinds and other light-diffusing measures may be wise.

If you are a writer, artist, or musician with winter SAD, you may be at your most productive and creative in spring or summer. The energy to create may elude you during both winter depressions and summer highs, when it's hard to focus.

Who Gets SAD?

In my clinical experience and in research studies, SAD is an equal-opportunity oppressor. People with SAD represent all races, ethnic groups, occupations, and ages. There are, however, some interesting patterns among those with seasonality. Check off all that apply to you:

☐ I am female.

☐ I live in the northern part of North America or Europe.

☐ My SAD symptoms started at puberty.

☐ I can see signs of SAD in family members and among previous generations of my family.

☐ I am a yo-yo dieter.

☐ I have fibromyalgia.

☐ My vocation/avocation is creative (art, music, poetry, drama).

☐ I have vision problems (see page 23).

☐ I feel more depressed the farther north I travel or live.

You may be surprised at this potpourri of diverse characteristics, and I am not implying that if you put them all together you will end up with the typical person with SAD. But each of these items *is* associated with the incidence of SAD, although in different ways, and knowing which of these factors is part of your SAD profile will help you understand more about your relationship with the seasons and what you can do to improve it.

- *Gender.* Although both men and women have SAD, it is *four times as common in women* as in men. We think this might be because the female sex hormones, estrogen and progesterone, are involved in SAD. That may explain why women are more seasonal than men during their 20s through 40s—the reproductive years—whereas after menopause men and women report roughly equal levels of seasonality. Also, many girls (but not boys) show a large increase in seasonal symptoms right after puberty.

- *Heritability.* Maybe your mother, a vibrant, energetic person at other times of year, has or had the same tendency you now have to curl up in front of the fire as often as possible in winter. Perhaps a grandparent, aunt, or uncle had a mood disorder of some kind, particularly one that worsened in winter. The rate of heritability among people with SAD varies widely, but if you can trace signs of SAD through your family roots, that may explain why you're experiencing some degree of SAD too. See Chapter 3 for more on genetic vulnerability to SAD.

Don't assume there's no SAD in your family if you find none in your parents or aunts and uncles. Go back another generation—or more. One of my patients was able to discern that many of the women in her generation had SAD even though each of them had a father with no active symptoms. Those fathers, however, all had mothers who, upon review by the family, likely did have SAD.

- *Eating habits and body weight.* People with SAD tend to overeat carbohydrate-rich foods—starches and sweets—when experiencing active SAD symptoms (usually the winter). So they gain weight, some of which they may lose in summer. Overeating around the winter holidays may not only be a result of a little innocent self-indulgence: it could be a sign of SAD. If you know this is part of your SAD pattern, you can take steps that will not only make the winter more bearable (feeling you have no control over your weight every year can certainly make you more depressed) but also improve your health in the years to come (because weight tends to pile up with each winter). There's evidence that people with SAD secrete too much insulin when they eat carbs. Too much insulin lowers blood sugar, producing a craving for more carbs—and a resulting weight gain (which makes you secrete even more insulin, and so on). So a vicious cycle ensues. All this results in an increased risk of diabetes and heart disease.

Myth Buster: People with SAD may be depressed and feel the need for comfort, but carbs are not a good solution. Nondepressed people tend to get drowsy when they eat carbs, but people with SAD tend to feel more energetic afterward. This may have something to do with the neurochemical serotonin, which increases in the brains of animals after they are fed carbohydrates. Low serotonin levels are associated with depression and with dark days, so people with SAD may feel a biological craving for breads and cakes on dark days because carbs restore the energy diminished by depression.

So what is the problem with eating carbs to boost energy? It helps only very briefly. Blood sugar levels will soon drop, making you lethargic and hungry all over again.

- *Latitude.* See the table on page 35, where data on the incidence of SAD at various latitudes has been compiled. SAD is particularly common in northern North America and Europe and seems to increase in severity or duration the farther north one goes. But note some interesting exceptions:

  - Icelanders don't have high rates of seasonality despite how far north they live. This relatively insular population may have evolved genes that protect them from SAD.
  - Low rates of SAD also appear among the Japanese and Chinese regardless of latitude, suggesting genetic protection among these groups too.

- *Fibromyalgia and other aches and pains.* If SAD makes you feel like you have the flu all winter, you're not alone. SAD often comes with all kinds of aches and pains.

- *Creativity.* The question of whether creativity is akin to madness has been raised since the time of Aristotle, and in much more recent years a few scientists have tried to answer it using modern psychiatric diagnoses. Most of the studies have been done on writers, and there is evidence that they often have mild forms of mood disorders (particularly bipolar disorder). What does this tell us about SAD and creativity? People with SAD often have a mild form of bipolar disorder with a seasonal pattern: depression in the winter and mania or

> *In the depth of winter, I finally learned that within me there lay an invincible summer.*
> —ALBERT CAMUS,
> RETURN TO TIPASA

hypomania in the summer. Creative writers often describe their productive periods in ways that SAD sufferers describe the euphoria of summer—as hypomania, a state of happy energy and optimism (as long as it stays in control).

At this point you have probably learned a few things about SAD and about your own experience with seasonality, and these discoveries may shed light on how aware of your problem you've been. I hope you feel motivated to learn more so that you can take whatever steps you need to feel better throughout the year.

You have SAD through no fault of your own, and you can feel better with the right APP: <u>a</u>wareness, <u>p</u>reparation, and <u>p</u>revention.

Chapter 2 will give you another opportunity to look at the pattern of your seasonality, along with the variability of your symptoms and particularly the impact of SAD on your life to further help you tackle the problem.

2

Your Seasonal Profile

★ KEY POINTS

What is the pattern of your seasonal problems?

How much do your symptoms vary with the seasons?

How much does SAD get in your way?

Be Aware

Chapter 1 gave you a chance to start looking clearly at your relationship with the seasons. I hope you now recognize SAD as a real disorder and your reactions to the change of seasons as a legitimate problem that deserves treatment. In this chapter you'll have an opportunity to continue your exploration, answering the three questions above and also determining how severe your symptoms are. All the information you gather will help you decide what type of help to pursue. The more you learn, the more power you have to prepare and prevent—and live happily and healthily year-round.

WHAT DOES YOUR SAD LOOK LIKE?

Back in 1984, my colleagues and I came up with a list of criteria by which to diagnose the disorder we named SAD. Over the next 15 years the psychiatric community became increasingly aware of the winter blues syndrome, and in the 2000 edition of its *Diagnostic and Statistical Manual of Mental Disorders* the American Psychiatric Association published its own, slightly different criteria. What's important is that the disorder is widely accepted today; exactly what is required to diagnose it is less relevant to you. For the purposes of feeling better all year, what you really need to know is whether, and to what extent, you have the core symptoms listed below and how severely those symptoms harm your life.

☀ *The Core Symptoms of SAD: Sound Familiar?*

- **Reduced energy**

- **Increasing eating, including carb cravings**

- **Weight gain**

- **Disturbed sleep**

- **Fatigue**

- **Lowered sex drive**

- **Thinking problems, including difficulty concentrating and processing information**

- **Mood problems, especially depression**

Even if you recognize some or all of the core symptoms as part of your winter doldrums, everybody's SAD is a little different. Knowing what your weak spots are will enable you to monitor and assess them so you can evaluate which suggestions offered in this book might help the most. With that in mind, on the facing page you'll find a quick questionnaire that can help you evaluate how seasonal you are.

Now let's see what your answers mean:

Your Seasonal Pattern (Question 1)

Check the appropriate box for how you filled out item H:

☐ **You feel worst in December, January, or February → You have winter pattern.**

☐ **You feel worst in July or August → You have summer pattern.**

☐ **You feel worst during Dec., Jan., or Feb. AND July or Aug. → You have summer–winter pattern.**

How Seasonal Are You?

Fill out the following information based on your experience over 3–5 years when you lived in a single climate—the more recent, the better. Fill in whatever circles apply.

1. *In what months do you . . .*

	J	F	M	A	M	J	J	A	S	O	N	D
A. Feel best												
B. Gain the most weight												
C. Socialize most												
D. Sleep least												
E. Eat most												
F. Lose most weight												
G. Socialize least												
H. Feel worst												
I. Eat least												
J. Sleep most												

2. *How much do the following change with the seasons? Circle whichever degree of change applies.*

	0 No change	1 Slight change	2 Moderate change	3 Marked change	4 Extremely marked change
A. Sleep length					
B. Social activity					
C. Mood (overall feeling of well-being)					
D. Weight					
E. Appetite					
F. Energy level					

3. *How big a problem are the changes you experience with the seasons?*

Mild	Moderate	Marked	Severe	Disabling

For now, set aside your answers to the other question 1 items. We'll get back to this shortly, and then you'll use this information again starting in Chapter 5.

The Severity of Your SAD and Its Impact on You: Your Global Seasonality Score (GSS) and Overall Severity Score (OSS) (Questions 2 and 3)

Add up the numbers for all the items in question 2 and check the box for your total global seasonality score:

☐ 8–10   →   **Moderate** seasonality

☐ 11–14   →   **Marked** seasonality

☐ 15–24   →   **Severe** seasonality

What degree of change you experience in each symptom (sleep, socializing, etc.) is also important. We'll come back to this information in Part II of this book.

On the surface, your global seasonality score (GSS) and overall severity score (OSS) should line up: Moderate seasonality should be a lesser problem for you, while marked seasonality is likely to pose a significant problem. Severe seasonality usually needs to be taken seriously. But it's not that simple; some people might find even mild seasonality disabling, and others might find moderate SAD manageable. A lot depends on your life circumstances. Say you work as a tour guide and you need to live in a northern climate because of your spouse's occupation. Even mild symptoms during the winter could make it very hard for you to drum up the energy, enthusiasm, and focus to guide tourists outdoors around your city or resort. Or say you are a schoolteacher who needs to get up at 6:30 A.M. Then even mild problems waking up could prove a major liability. On the other hand, you could conceivably have a total GSS of 16 and not consider it too much of a liability—maybe you don't have to have a job and you don't have family obligations and can virtually hibernate during the winter. Given the hectic lives most people lead, however, a GSS of 16 will usually be a liability. But you will find that the less stressful your circumstances, the lower your score will go, and vice versa. So if you scored a 16 while working as a tour guide in the North, you might have difficulty functioning, but then let's say you suddenly win the lottery—now your GSS goes down because you're not subject to the same stresses.

🔆 **It's pretty typical for people living in the northern hemisphere to sleep and eat more and gain weight in the winter. That's not enough to indicate you have SAD.**

It's the whole picture, reflected by the GSS, that is a better clue as to whether you likely have SAD.

|▲| SCIENCE

Which group tends to have the most severe SAD?

☐ Men in their mid-20s

☐ Women in their early 20s

☐ Men ages 50–60

☐ Women in their late 30s

☐ Senior citizens

☐ Children

In a study colleagues and I did at NIMH, women in their late 30s had the most severe SAD. There was less evidence that men's seasonality changed with age, and in women SAD became milder after age 40.

WHERE IS SAD A PROBLEM FOR YOU?

Now that you have some sense of how seasonal you are and how big a problem SAD can become for you, let's look at some important specific areas of functioning that can become disrupted in the winter (or in summer for those with a summer pattern).

Work

Check off each item that represents your experience during the time of year you feel worst (try to think of the last 3 years).

☐ I get tired much earlier in the workday and feel exhausted on my way home.

☐ I really don't care about my job at all and can't make the decisions I need to make.

☐ I miss a lot of work and end up using vacation time after using up my sick days and personal days.

☐ I had to quit my job. I just couldn't get up and go in anymore.

☐ People at work were getting upset with me—and vice versa.

Recreational Activities

Check off each item that represents your experience during the time of year you feel worst (try to think of the last 3 years).

☐ I can't play tennis [golf, basketball, etc.] or work out to my usual level. I just feel weak and tired.

☐ My latest craft project ends up sitting in the basement gathering dust, half finished. I'm not interested in it anymore.

☐ I used to go hiking [skiing, camping, folk dancing, etc.] every weekend, but now I go about once a month, at most.

☐ I quit the team [club, class, etc.].

It's no surprise that work and other activities demand commitment, energy, and focus, no matter what your occupation. All of these capacities are compromised by SAD. The more items you checked above, the more severe your SAD may be. Three problems may be at work: changes in cognition (thinking ability), energy level, and physical/health issues. The more depressed people are (with SAD and other types of depression), the more slowly they think, the less they can concentrate, the harder they find it to make decisions. Meanwhile, they may feel fatigued or drained and have stomachaches and loss of appetite, backaches and headaches, and general malaise. No wonder it's hard to work *or* play.

⚗ SCIENCE

A brain-wave study of the ability to respond to a visual stimulus showed that attention increases in those with SAD following light therapy. In other words, disruptions in mental functioning that you notice at work (or at play) is only temporary and can be reversed with treatment. So with light comes hope for better mood and functioning.

Relationships

Check off each item that represents your experience during the time of year you feel worst (try to think of the last 3 years).

☐ I don't really feel like going to parties or other social events, but I usually keep doing it.

☐ I turn down a fair number of invitations and just stay home on my free time.

☐ When I must be around people, I have to be coaxed into conversation and find it hard to smile and joke with others, even my own family.

☐ My spouse/partner says I'm totally withdrawn and is worried about me. My kids keep asking me what's wrong. Some of my friends have stopped calling altogether.

The same things that interfere with work and leisure pursuits can hamper interpersonal relationships. But because these activities interact with one another, mood problems that emerge as pessimism and feeling ill can make other problems worse. People with SAD sometimes feel anxious as well as depressed, which adds to the general distress.

🔆 **If you have any doubt about how seasonality may be affecting your relationships, ask your spouse/partner or other close relative or friend. Others who care about you will be glad to be invited to let you know how your depression appears to them— and what its impact is on your relationship. And they are often surprisingly good observers.**

Sleep

Check off each item that represents your experience during the time of year you feel worst (try to think of the last 3 years).

☐ I can't seem to get enough sleep.

☐ A "short" nap will end up lasting for hours.

☐ I have difficulty waking up in the morning.

☐ My sleep is disrupted.

We spend about a third of our lives sleeping. So if our sleep is disturbed, so are our lives. We need good sleep to feel refreshed. Just as sleep is often affected by SAD, daytime energy and vitality are affected by the quality of the sleep we get.

Total score on seasonality in different domains of life (number of items checked): _____

Your total score on the domain questions could be up to 17, depending on how many items you checked. The higher your total, the more severe—and pervasive in your life—your seasonality is likely to be. And you're not alone; when people in the northern parts of the United States were surveyed, **about one-quarter of them said they had problems with the changing seasons** (taking into account all patterns and levels of severity of seasonality).

|▲| SCIENCE

Do You Find Yourself Self-Medicating in the Season That Causes You Trouble?

Many people who have SAD tend to self-medicate.

- ☐ *Do you overeat the types of food that you tend to indulge less in during other seasons—chocolate, cookies, and candy—not to mention bread and pasta?* Although these generally tend to sedate people, those with SAD get a short, temporary energizing boost from them.

- ☐ *Do you consume more caffeinated beverages than usual?* Some people with SAD report drinking many more cups of coffee, tea, or caffeinated soda or energy drinks than they do during the other seasons because they need the caffeine to stay awake or alert.

- ☐ *Are you drinking more alcohol at this time of year?* People may feel better temporarily after a couple of drinks (or a lot more), but there will usually be a backlash: alcohol is known to aggravate the symptoms of depression. In those with SAD it's hard to tell whether drinking is the *result* of depression (trying to "drown your sorrows"), the cause of depressed feelings, or both (in which case a vicious cycle ensues).

- ☐ *Do you smoke?* I have seen those with seasonal symptoms take up tobacco and/or marijuana in their difficult season, despite its lack of appeal the rest of the year.

THE BOTTOM LINE:
WHAT DO MY SCORES TELL ME TO DO?

First consider your global seasonality score (GSS):

☐ *My global seasonality score was 0–7 in the "How Seasonal Are You?" questionnaire.* You don't have any significant problem with seasonality. *However,* you've read this far in this book, which must mean that the changes in season are a downer, at least to some extent. Maybe you just don't feel as good, overall, during winter as at other times of year and you'd like to change that. Perhaps one season of the year finds you less creative or productive, working harder at your job or in your relationships than before. It may be worth trying a little extra environmental light, through a light box or the other measures suggested in Chapter 8 and see if they help.

☐ *My global seasonality score was 8–10 in the "How Seasonal Are You?" questionnaire.* You're definitely experiencing noticeable problems, and you probably have what we call moderate SAD. You might not qualify for a clinical diagnosis, but you could use some self-help. You'll find plenty of it throughout this book. Read Chapters 4–6 to identify the best options for you and then use the corresponding chapters later in the book to monitor your progress with those remedies and see if you can rid yourself of *all* seasonal symptoms, as I do (most of the time).

☐ *My global seasonality score was higher than 11 in the "How Seasonal Are You?" questionnaire.* Your seasonality is probably at least moderate in severity, and you might enjoy faster, more thorough improvement if you consulted a professional.

Your GSS measures the severity of your seasonality, which will generally equate to how big a problem these symptoms are for you. But as mentioned earlier, a lot depends on your life circumstances and level of stress during the seasons that bring you down, so take the extent that seasonal changes cause problems in your life into account as well.

☐ *I checked off "mild" on question 3 of the "How Seasonal Are You?" questionnaire.* Whether to treat your SAD will be mostly a quality-of-life matter. If you checked off only a few areas of functioning where SAD is a problem for you during your worst time(s) of year, you may decide to take minor measures to ease symptoms and see how it goes. Chapters 4–6 will give you a preliminary idea of what might be easiest and simplest for you, and then Part II will give you the information you need to apply your choices.

☐ *I checked off "moderate" on question 3 of the "How Seasonal Are You?" questionnaire.* You should definitely treat your symptoms so as not to suffer functionally in important areas of your life. If you noticed particular problems in certain areas of functioning, that information may point you to the best remedies to try (introduced in Chapter 4).

☐ *I checked off "marked," "severe," or "disabling" on question 3 of the "How Seasonal Are You?" questionnaire.* If you feel the problems that seasonality causes you are marked, it's probably best to check in with a doctor, who can help you decide on a course of action and then help you follow through with treatment as needed. If seasonal changes are a severe or disabling problem for you, and you checked off the majority of areas of functioning as domains in which SAD affects you, definitely see your doctor.

🔆 *You should definitely seek medical help if:*

- *You really can't function well.* You can't get to work, produce at work, or get along with coworkers; you're withdrawing from family and friends; you're letting go of important responsibilities, like taking care of your finances or skipping medical checkups.

- *You feel significantly depressed.* You feel very sad or are crying frequently; you feel worthless, guilty, or pessimistic.

- *Life doesn't feel worthwhile to you.*

- *Your physical functioning has changed dramatically.* You're sleeping much longer, can't seem to drag yourself out of bed, feel exhausted during the day, or your eating and weight are out of control.

🧪 SCIENCE

Your doctor might consider the following diagnoses, in addition to SAD, because they can mimic the symptoms:

Hypothyroidism: An underactive thyroid can mimic SAD by making you feel tired and intolerant of the cold, and it's usually easily corrected with thyroid hormone pills.

Hypoglycemia: Low blood sugar can make you feel weak and lightheaded and also crave sweets. The symptoms can usually be prevented through avoidance of sugar and a diet made up of proteins, vegetables, fruits, and legumes (which may be a good idea anyway).

☐ *I identified a definite seasonal pattern in question 1 in the "How Seasonal Are You?" questionnaire.* Some of the suggestions in this book will be of benefit no matter what your seasonal pattern, and some will apply only to winter depression or one of the other patterns. In the next four chapters you'll have a chance to put together everything you have now learned about your own seasonal profile so that you can pick the best treatment options for you, whether your problems occur in winter, summer, spring, fall, or a combination.

Remember, if you have SAD, you can feel better!

3

What's Making You Feel
So SAD?

Distress that persists or keeps returning eventually becomes impossible to ignore. In Chapter 2 you started to look more closely at your seasonal distress, answering questions about what's going on, whether it's "real," and whether it needs to be addressed. As a result you may feel a little more accepting of having the legitimate problem called SAD—and a little closer to solving it. Now it would be only natural to ask "Why me?"

That's an excellent question, because it has concrete answers that can point you to treatments and remedies that will help.

In many fields of medicine today—mental and physical—causation is generally viewed as multifaceted. When we look for the causes of an illness or disorder, we look to both internal and external processes:

- *Biology*—physiological conditions and predispositions

- *Psychology*—your thoughts, emotions, and behavior

- *Environment (stress)*—your physical surroundings, your daily routine (at home and work), and your relationships

As important as considering all three factors mentioned above is understanding how they operate together. Although scientists often try to gain an overall understanding of a particular illness, the best treatment plan for any individual person relies on an understanding of the particulars of the individual in question, meaning *you*.

In the case of SAD, the fabric of causes is woven out of:

- Your genetic tendencies

- How much light you're getting and when and how you're getting it

- Your stress level (or the amount of stress in your life)

Your brain's biochemistry is the ultimate arena in which these various factors cause SAD. Your gender, genetic tendencies, and even the effects of light influence the chemical interactions in the brain that in turn create seasonal symptoms. Likewise, environmental factors influence brain chemistry. The most important environmental cause of SAD is your **exposure to light.** How far do you live from the equator? How much light is available in your home? How much light is in your workspace? Your answers to these questions will give you important clues about your overall light exposure. **Stress** is the third major factor in causing SAD, and that depends both on what is happening to you and your resources for handling it.

How do you think these three factors cause your own seasonality? Jot any ideas you have here:

_____

_____

_____

_____

_____

_____

_____

_____

YOUR BRAIN'S BIOCHEMISTRY

The emotional, mental, and physical disturbances of SAD are strongly governed by the light registered in the brain through the physical feature of the eyes, but other factors also contribute to SAD. For example: (1) gender and the effects of the female hormones mentioned in Chapter 2; (2) your family history, operating via genetic variants that affect neurochemicals and the eye's involvement in circadian rhythms; and (3) melatonin, a hormone centrally involved in circadian rhythms that may be important to our understanding of SAD. Light intimately affects all these processes.

Be Aware

Are Female Hormones Making You SAD?

Circle Yes or No:

Do you regularly have premenstrual syndrome symptoms (food cravings, fluid retention, irritability, abdominal cramps) in the week or two before your period?	**Yes**	**No**
Do these symptoms remind you of your SAD symptoms?	**Yes**	**No**
Do you have PMS exclusively or more frequently in the winter than the rest of the year?	**Yes**	**No**
Did the onset of your SAD symptoms coincide (roughly) with your first periods?	**Yes**	**No**

If you answered yes to two or three of these questions, your seasonality may in fact be related to estrogen and progesterone. If you're close to menopause, the reduction in female hormones may improve your SAD symptoms along with your PMS. But it may also mean that treatments for SAD could improve your PMS!

Did You Inherit SAD?

In the fairly recent past, many psychological disturbances were considered a product of environment, particularly problematic parenting or other traumas that occurred in early childhood. Today the position that mental illnesses are just as biological as physiological problems like heart disease has gained a lot of support. The brain is, after all, according to one scientist, "the organ of the mind. Where else could [mental illness] be if not in the brain?"*

This perspective has given rise to a lot of research into genetic vulnerability of chronic illnesses, including so-called mental illnesses like SAD. If the problem lies

---

*Eric Kandel, MD, Columbia University professor and Nobel laureate, quoted by Kirsten Weir, American Psychological Association, "The Roots of Mental Illness," June 2012, Vol. 43, No. 6, *www.apa.org/monitor/2012/06/roots.aspx*.

in the biology of the brain, what is driving the brain to produce the symptoms of SAD? Apparently genetics do play a role. Studies of heritability often focus on identical twins because they have virtually identical genes. In at least one large study of twins, genetics were definitely seen to be a factor in the degree to which people's mood and behavior vary with the seasons.

Do you think you could have a family history of SAD? In many cases genes express themselves in different ways in different individuals within the same family, so sometimes people with SAD find that even though only a few individuals in their family tree had SAD per se, many more had depression or some related mood disorder. Identifying a family history of SAD or other depression *may* give you valuable treatment information, because treatments that work for one member of a family often work for others. Beyond that, though, discovering that you might have inherited SAD reinforces your understanding of the biological basis of seasonality—*and the fact that having SAD isn't your fault.* If you're interested in investigating your own family history of mood problems in general and SAD in particular, fill out the form on the next page. Feel free to copy it (or download it from *www.guilford.com/rosenthal3-forms*) if you need more space or if you want to use it another time in the future.

There are no hard-and-fast rules for determining how many relatives with SAD or a related illness constitutes a genetic predisposition, but obviously, the larger the number, the greater your probable genetic vulnerability. An example (without names filled in so that you can see the relationships) is shown on page 42.

The family tree on page 43 was drawn by Hannah, who at age 40 has been noticing SAD symptoms since she was about 13. Her own daughter, age 14, is starting to show signs of depression, although she is not yet sure they are associated with any particular season. Hannah has a sister who has exhibited signs of hypomania and depression (bipolar II disorder), although she hasn't been diagnosed, and another sister who definitely shares Hannah's SAD history. Their mother never knew to call her winter blues SAD, but when the core symptoms were described, she and her family members agreed that she seemed to have had many of them over the years. Mom's brother says he felt pretty down "on and off" over the years of his adult life but hasn't noticed much more than that. Hannah's maternal grandparents died long ago, and no one can remember any particular signs of depression. Hannah's father is sure his mother had SAD, describing her as "practically hibernating" starting in December, which he remembers putting a damper on the holiday fun year after year.

Hannah could have come by SAD partly through a genetic link with both her mother and her paternal grandmother. Note the evidence of depression and mood disorders among both men and women in the family, but more in the women, and SAD only in the women. This reflects the greater incidence of all these disorders in women than in men and shows the potential for a genetic predisposition to be passed down through a generation by the males, to be expressed in the next generation, predominantly in the females. This family tree also shows that people can

Your SAD Family Tree

Be Aware

Gather as much information as you can on your relatives over the last couple of generations (or further into the past). Fill in the names of your relatives in the appropriate boxes, adding ovals for additional females and rectangles for additional males. Then enter what you discovered about the presence of mood disorders, depression, and SAD by using either colored pencils/markers/crayons or initials, as follows:

Mood disorder (unspecified, either some form of depression or bipolar disorder or even chronic general "moodiness"): Purple or M

Depression (any form): Blue or D

SAD: Gray or S

If you know the person was diagnosed with a clinical disorder, put an asterisk in the box. For undiagnosed problems nonetheless recognized by you or other family members, omit the asterisk.

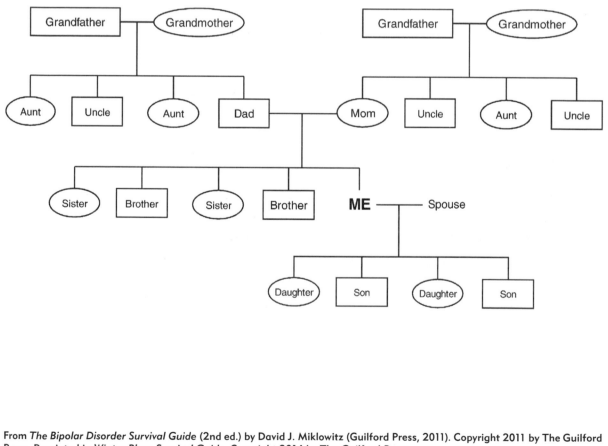

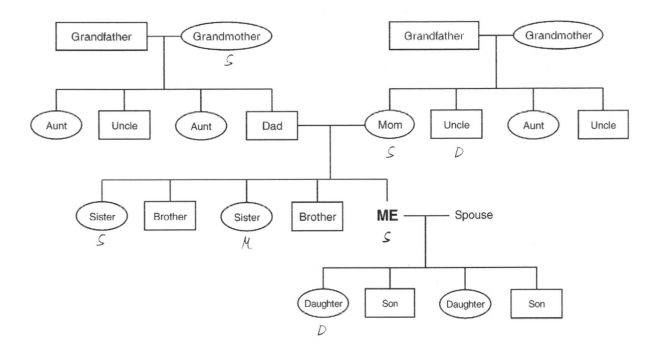

and often do experience symptoms of illnesses without being diagnosed or treated, which may obscure the genetic association.

Knowing your genetic history can help spare you and later generations of your family from feeling unwarranted shame and from suffering without the treatment they need.

What Does It Mean If You Have No Family History of SAD?

SAD does run in families, and most people with SAD have at least one close relative with a history of depression (often SAD). But the fact that you have no family history doesn't mean *you* don't have SAD. Maybe there's a genetic variant lurking somewhere among your ancestors but concealed by the sands of time or by something that exerted a protective effect. Maybe no one in your family was aware of—or admitted to—having seasonal problems. Or maybe you are the first member of your family to have SAD—a true original!

SCIENCE

How Brain Chemistry Varies in SAD

Everything that we do and everything that happens in our bodies (digestion, breathing, heartbeat, etc.) is dictated by the brain, which operates through an intricate network of cells (neurons) that communicate through chemical messengers called *neurotransmitters*. It is likely that three major neurotransmitter systems operate differently in those who have SAD than in people without SAD symptoms.

Here are a few things we know about these three neurotransmitters—serotonin, dopamine, and norepinephrine—and SAD:

- Serotonin in a part of the brain that governs eating, sleeping, and biological rhythms (the hypothalamus) drops significantly in the winter.

- Serotonin levels in the blood vary directly with the amount of sunlight present on any particular day.

- Brain serotonin levels rise when people with SAD eat carb-rich foods.

- Dopamine fuels pleasure and energy. It also contributes to our ability to regulate body temperature and to the functioning of the eyes, which are the portals through which light influences the brain.

- Norepinephrine governs the secretion of melatonin, a hormone that may be important in the development of SAD (see below). Norepinephrine also regulates alertness, which is less acute than normal in people with SAD.

LIGHT AND SAD

We know the seasons affect us largely through the changes they bring in the amount of daily sunlight. But we can also learn a lot about the causes of SAD by looking at exactly how we react biologically to the daily cycle of night and day—our circadian rhythms.

When light enters our eyes, it sets off a sequence of neurochemical events that can switch off melatonin secretion. In animals, this can regulate energy level, drive to reproduce, and appetite. Could these neurochemical effects, acting via melatonin, also be important in SAD? We and other researchers have set out trying to answer this question.

Melatonin: A Curfew for the Parting Day

The hormone melatonin signals that dusk is falling by being secreted in the brain at night and receding at dawn. While we don't know exactly what physiological responses it triggers, we know it is a biological marker for our experience of day and night. Now picture our cave-dwelling predecessors, lacking artificial light, lying quietly in darkness for 14 hours a night in the winter. Those long nights resulted in correspondingly longer periods of melatonin secretion, compared to the shorter nights of summer. In modern times our brains still secrete melatonin during the dark hours, but because we now have artificial light, we experience the shorter period of melatonin secretion even during winter. At least that applies to people who do *not* have SAD. Those who *do* have SAD, however, secrete melatonin for a longer duration during winter nights. It is as if they are not "seeing" artificial (low-intensity) light from a melatonin point of view.

💡 *Does SAD Represent a Primitive Form of Sleep Deprivation?*

People with SAD may feel tired and cranky during the shorter days of winter because of their extended secretion of melatonin: *This hormone may be telling them they are supposed to be in bed.*

🧪 SCIENCE

Reinforcing the possible connection between melatonin and SAD is the fact that one of the genetic variants found to be connected to SAD involves *melanopsin*, a pigment found in cells of the retina that changes chemically when it absorbs light, sending signals to the brain that affect certain circadian rhythm functions, including the suppression of melatonin secretion.

In animals melatonin also seems to regulate the drive to reproduce seasonally. This seasonal regulation is important because it enables animals to be sexually active and conceive at those times that will ensure that the young are born in spring, when the weather is hospitable and food is more plentiful. Could melatonin be involved in sex drive in humans too? Quite possibly—since it is involved in regulating female reproductive hormones and thereby in menstruation. Some women with SAD actually stop menstruating in the winter, and a core feature of SAD (see Chapter 2) is lowered libido.

Be Aware

Is a Genetic Variant in Melatonin Secretion Making You SAD?

Circle **Yes** or **No**:

In the winter, do you often feel that if you could just sleep as long as you want, you'd feel fine?	**Yes**	**No**
Do you find yourself rarely interested in sex during winter?	**Yes**	**No**

Does the pattern of your menstrual periods change during winter?	**Yes**	**No**
Have you noticed development or worsening of SAD symptoms following a move farther north?	**Yes**	**No**
Have you noticed development or worsening of SAD symptoms after moving from a bright residence or workplace to a dark one?	**Yes**	**No**
Do you notice SAD-like symptoms during a long stretch of gloomy weather, regardless of the season?	**Yes**	**No**

Be Aware

Is a Biological Variant in Serotonin or Other Neurotransmitters Making You SAD?

Circle Yes or No:

Have you ever taken an antidepressant that affects serotonin and found that your SAD symptoms were alleviated?	**Yes**	**No**
Do you often eat cookies or candy and feel energized for a short time afterward?	**Yes**	**No**

STRESS AND SAD

So many things can cause stress—a difficult relationship, too many responsibilities, too little money, illness in oneself or others, and much more.

Be Aware

Check off all of the following that causes stress in your life:

- ☐ Marital/relationship conflict
- ☐ Child-rearing issues
- ☐ Caregiving for parents or siblings
- ☐ Loneliness/isolation
- ☐ Friendship difficulties
- ☐ Financial problems
- ☐ Conflicts with coworkers or employers
- ☐ Too many work responsibilities
- ☐ Feeling underappreciated by family, friends, or colleagues

☐ Legal problems

☐ Chores/home maintenance

☐ Transportation difficulties

☐ Illness or injury (your own)

☐ Illness or injury (in someone close to you)

☐ Substance use

☐ Poor diet

☐ Lack of exercise

☐ Uncomfortable living quarters

☐ Schoolwork

☐ Sleep problems

☐ Pessimism

☐ Perfectionism

☐ Unrealistic expectations

☐ Anger

☐ Guilt

☐ Unemployment

☐ Loss of a loved one

☐ Dangerous environment

☐ Moving to a new community

☐ Getting married or divorced

Obviously there are many other possibilities to consider that are aspects of your personal, financial, occupational, emotional, social, and spiritual life. These are just common examples.

Stress can also cause many problems, physical and mental—SAD being one of them. As stresses pile one on top of the other, it is easy to feel overloaded and overwhelmed. Check off signs of stress overload that you're experiencing or have experienced in the past:

☐ Feeling on edge, like you're always poised for fight or flight

☐ Having chronic pain or discomfort, like a headache, backache, or stomach distress

☐ Being short tempered, easy to anger

☐ Having difficulty concentrating

☐ Making decisions you (and others) later question

☐ Having memory problems

☐ Worrying incessantly

☐ Feeling alone and isolated

☐ Feeling flushed, with heart racing

☐ Catching a lot of colds

☐ Needing alcohol, cigarettes, or drugs to relax

☐ Losing sleep

☐ Eating too much or too little

Here, too, these are just some of the signs of being overloaded and overwhelmed. Any lasting negative change in how you feel physically or emotionally or in your thinking ability may be a sign of excess stress.

Stresses vary from season to season. Because stress makes SAD symptoms worse, an increase in stress from one winter to the next can catch you by surprise. For example, Susan is a young mother who usually managed to get through the winter quite well even though she felt a little less energetic, a bit down, and gained a few pounds. But one January, when she ended up largely responsible for getting her father through a serious illness, she sank into a much deeper depression. Although this additional burden on top of her usual parenting duties and a part-time job would get anyone down, Susan felt much better in April, even though her responsibilities remained.

Susan demonstrated an important formula:

Stress + mild SAD = BAD SAD

Once the vicious cycle kicks in, it's hard to reverse until the spring. The trick is to try to catch the problem as early as possible. A much better formula than the one demonstrated by Susan's recent winter is:

SAD's Vicious Cycle

Stress can trigger SAD symptoms or make them worse. But when someone has SAD, stresses feel worse. That can make you more stressed out than at other times of the year. Because of this vicious circle, which can make you feel like you're being dragged down more and more, it is so important to pay attention to identifying sources of stress in your life and finding ways to prevent and resolve them.

Treat SAD soon + Fix stress = MUCH less distress

Protecting Yourself from Chronic Stress

Because stress can be much harder on you in the winter when you have SAD, it's worth avoiding. Another reason to avoid stress is that chronic stress can have cumulative negative effects on cardiovascular health, blood sugar levels, and even muscles and bones. Solution? The relaxation response (Chapter 12), which shuts off the secretion of cortisol, the so-called stress hormone, protecting your health and preventing your SAD from worsening.

Be Aware

Is Stress a Problem for You and Your Seasonality?

Circle **Yes** or **No:**

Have you ever noticed your seasonal symptoms worsening when a stressful event occurred?	**Yes**	**No**
Do you suffer frequent headaches, stomachaches, muscle tension, wakefulness, indigestion or lack of appetite at all times of year?	**Yes**	**No**
Do you think you spend a lot of time worrying about the future or rehashing the past?	**Yes**	**No**

There are numerous ways to manage stress—managing your time, meditating, ensuring that your daily life includes pleasant activities, learning progressive relaxation. These are explained in full in Part II. For now, take a moment to think about the stresses that affect your life and what you might be able to do to limit their damaging effects.

HOW CAUSES INFORM TREATMENT

The next few chapters will give you a chance to link what you've learned so far about your own SAD with solutions and preventive measures you can take, either via self-help or with the assistance of a health practitioner. What causes an illness can provide valuable information about how to

Heading Off Stress

Prevent

What are your current stresses, or what stresses do you anticipate next winter (or whatever is your season of risk)? Next to each item, there is room to write potential remedies or antidotes for these stresses. This might include remedies that have worked in the past or those that are listed in this book. Be sure to return to this list when you're done reading this book (don't worry; I'll remind you) so that you can see what new SAD-busting tricks you have learned as a result of your reading. Don't worry if the same remedy appears more than once.

Stress	Remedies/Antidotes

resolve it, but as you've now seen, several factors are involved in causing SAD. Therefore the relationship between cause and treatment is not always clear. In fact, the most important conclusion you can draw from understanding what causes SAD is that there are multiple causes, and a combination of treatments is almost always most effective.

For example, if you are sharply aware that when daylight wanes early in fall you feel as if you're slipping into a fog, extra light is likely to help you. Light therapy, described in Chapter 7, is powerfully effective, but bumping up environmental light and even taking a winter vacation to a sunny place (Chapter 8) can help too. Light therapy can also be a big help if you're a woman and have noticed a similarity between how you feel during premenstrual days of the month and when you experience SAD symptoms. Studies have shown that those who suffer from PMS and SAD often find both problems eased with light.

Now picture adding stress management—shortening your winter to-do list, learning meditation or progressive relaxation, adding pleasant activities to your daily routine (Chapters 9, 12, and 13). Your SAD Solution APP just got a surge of power.

One more idea (although you'll find *many* more in the rest of this book): If you're often hit by waves of self-blame, immobilized by pessimism, or tortured by guilt over not being at your best during your season of risk, consider a mental tune-up using the proven techniques of cognitive-behavioral therapy (see Chapter 14). They can help free you to seek the help you need, to focus on what's important, and to look toward a sunny horizon throughout the year.

Prevent   **The bottom line: Come at SAD from every angle available to you.**

The next chapter will show you how to choose what might offer you the most relief but also be easiest to incorporate into your own lifestyle and personal preferences. That's your SAD Solution APP-T.

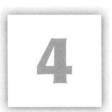

4

Identifying the Best Treatments for You

Understanding SAD can transform the way you travel through the seasons every year. If you read Chapter 3, you may already be noticing a shift in your understanding—or at least imagining the possibilities as to how your worst season can become . . . well, not so bad.

Becoming aware that the energy drain you experience in fall is caused by your brain's reaction to the waning daylight may lead you to seek out new sources of bright light. Maybe you'll start planning ahead for a February vacation in the sun. You might even stop blaming yourself for being unable to shake off the post-holiday blues now that you know what's behind them. Realizing that beating yourself up for having difficulty getting things done during winter does you no good (in fact, it has always made you feel worse) is an excellent start. The next step is being realistic about what you *can* do. That helps you think differently about yourself and your world. Your expectations begin to change. You feel a little more in control. Hope begins to stir—and you feel better. Maybe winter doesn't have to control how you feel. You can use this new understanding and the happier mood that comes with it to take a chance and experiment with even more ideas for pushing SAD into the background of your life. This is just one illustration of how understanding can lead you down a new path toward feeling better in spite of SAD.

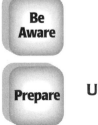

Be Aware **Understanding opens your eyes.**

Prepare **Understanding changes your outlook and drives new behavior.**

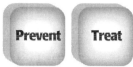

Understanding breeds solutions.

At the end of Chapter 3, I advocated coming at SAD from every angle available to you. The illustration above shows why that approach tends to work: extra light reverses depression, and when you feel better, you have more of the personal resources you need to put stress management methods in place. This phenomenon also illustrates an important principle to keep in mind throughout your journey toward well-being:

SYNERGY produces ENERGY.

With light therapy *and* stress management methods in place, your capacity to pursue even more improvements in SAD symptoms keeps growing. You're going to get geometrically greater benefits from combining treatment strategies, because typically each tack you take is going to boost the effectiveness of the others. Add light and you lift a veil that lightens the effort to start exercising or resist food cravings. Challenge automatic negative thoughts and unhelpful beliefs and you make it easier to drop the *shoulds* that will do their best to add back the stress you've been reducing. Start exercising and avoid alcohol and tobacco and you automatically reduce stress while getting physically healthier. These are just a few examples. The synergistic effects of taking multiple treatment approaches will conserve your energy and increase the overall antidepressant effects you reap. Therefore, even though it makes sense to know what might help you the most, and what type of treatment you might want to start with, your goal will be to come at SAD from at least the first two angles in the box below and possibly the third (in the form of medication).

In this chapter you'll add to your understanding of cause by getting an overview of the treatments available to you. Knowing a little about what each treatment can do for you, how you can access it, and what the pros and cons are will give you an idea of exactly what you might like to try and how you might use the remedy,

---

The Three Targets for Treating SAD

1. *Your light and your world*

2. *Your mind and your way of thinking*

3. *Your brain chemistry*

---

how effective it is in fighting SAD, and some things you should know about opting for this kind of treatment. This is helpful preparation for making the best use of the chapters in Part II so that you can prevent symptoms as much as possible and treat those you can't prevent.

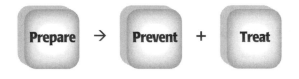

YOUR LIGHT AND YOUR WORLD

The principle behind light therapy is glaringly simple: this treatment replaces the missing light that is causing your SAD. The most effective, most reliable way to get light therapy is by using a light fixture designed for this purpose, although you can also try exposing yourself to as much outdoor daylight as possible and brightening your indoor environment. All of these methods will provide light on a daily basis (although outdoor light varies with factors beyond your control, like weather conditions). You might also supplement these methods with winter trips to a sunnier, warmer region. Finally, if your SAD proves treatment resistant, you might consider the more drastic measure of moving to a latitude closer to the equator.

Light Fixtures (See Chapter 7)

Light fixtures come in various forms, and there is also a nifty piece of equipment called a dawn simulator that can give you an artificial sunrise to help you wake up.

Pros

- Often the only treatment needed
- Easy to use
- Suitable for self-help
- Reliable equipment is available
- Best results from early-morning use, so benefits may be noticed all day at work

Cons

- Optimal use (type of fixture, position, duration, time of day) requires some experimentation
- Initial investment of $100–250
- Needs to be scheduled and committed to: For most people, skipping more than 1 day of treatment causes a return of symptoms

- Can benefit PMS as well as SAD

- Exposure can easily be increased or decreased as needed

- Often act rapidly—within 2 to 4 days

- Unwieldy to travel with light boxes

- Can cause side effects, although they are usually minor and often stop in a couple of weeks

Remember: Light therapy and dawn simulation can often be used together to excellent effect. I also almost always recommend putting stress management methods in place at the same time as light therapy, although some people may find stress management more effective once they've received some mood-boosting benefit from light therapy.

How interested are you in trying light therapy (on a scale of 1–10)? _____

How interested are you in trying a dawn simulator (on a scale of 1–10)? _____

If you're interested in light therapy, how could you plan to get it?

☐ Read Chapter 7 to learn all about light therapy.

☐ Research light fixtures online.

☐ Talk to your doctor about any questions you have.

☐ Invest in a light fixture immediately.

☐ Invest in a dawn simulator immediately or after trying a regular light fixture.

☐ Figure out when you could schedule regular light therapy and where you could do it.

☐ Other: _____

Adding Light to Your Current Surroundings (See Chapter 8)

You can brighten your home in a variety of ways, from increasing the sunlight streaming in to installing more lighting to redecorating. Adding light to your workspace may be more difficult since you won't necessarily be able to modify it, but a lot may be negotiable, depending on whether you are "out" about your SAD. (And some light fixtures look like desk lamps and won't be recognized as "therapeutic.")

Pros	Cons
• Flexible way to increase light that can suit your aesthetics	• Limited choices if you don't own the space
• Benefits from one-time efforts	• Rarely sufficient as treatment for all but the mildest cases of SAD
	• Minimal benefits if you spend a lot of time moving from place to place during the day

How interested are you in brightening your home (on a scale of 1–10)? _____

How interested are you in brightening your workplace (on a scale of 1–10)? _____

If you're interested in brightening your environment, what do you think you might do?

☐ **Read Chapter 8.**

☐ **Write up a list of quick and easy changes to make to add light at home.**

☐ **Figure out how to get more light at work.**

☐ **Talk to your boss about getting more light into your work area.**

☐ **Other:** _____

Getting Away to Sunnier Locales (See Chapter 8)

Almost everyone enjoys a break from winter chill and gloom, so January and February vacations to the Caribbean and other warm climates closer to the equator are perennially popular. For people with SAD, they offer more than relaxing leisure. Even a week away, with long, bright days, can be a huge relief and can sometimes make the subsequent weeks of winter easier, as you build on the boost the trip gives you. Another option is, instead of heading south, to go skiing. The mountains of the western United States tend to have sunny days year-round, and the combination of the bright sun and its reflection off the snow can lessen the winter blues.

A more drastic getaway is relocation, which can help those who really can't find a way to live comfortably with SAD where they currently reside.

Pros	Cons

Pros

- Even if the light-therapy benefit doesn't last, anticipating and then building on the effects of a winter vacation can ease depression.

- Relocating might eliminate the need for any treatment at all (although typically people still need to treat their SAD in the new place).

- More favorable climates, either on vacation or as permanent moves, usually increase healthy outdoor recreation and exercise generally.

Cons

- The benefits of vacations might not last and therefore might not be worth the cost.

- Moving to a new place can be stressful in and of itself, which can exacerbate depression.

- The new location may have different problems you haven't anticipated.

- A location that's warm and sunny in winter may be *too* hot and sunny in summer, causing a different seasonal problem.

How interested are you in trying to take winter vacations (on a scale of 1–10)? _____

How interested are you in relocating (on a scale of 1–10)? _____

If you're interested in getting more light by taking a vacation or moving, what do you think you would do?

☐ **Read Chapter 8.**

☐ **Start researching winter vacation possibilities.**

☐ **Think about the pros and cons of making a permanent move.**

☐ **Other:** _____

YOUR MIND AND YOUR WAY OF THINKING

SAD is certainly not all in your head. But the way you think, and the way you behave based on your thoughts and feelings, has a lot to do with how severely you are impaired by a tendency toward seasonality. Light exerts biochemical effects in the brain, and so does shifting your way of thinking. Your options for reducing stress and taking a "mind over mood" attitude (Chapters 9–14) are wide ranging and can fit a variety of needs.

Acceptance (See Chapter 9)

It's important to come to terms with having SAD, but that's easier said than done. Many people with SAD have an ongoing struggle with acceptance: they continue to blame themselves for having the illness and have trouble holding on to the fact that the limitations they experience in their season(s) of depression are not their fault. Unfortunately, lack of acceptance not only makes them feel worse but also creates roadblocks to treatment. Accepting that you have a legitimate illness and have the right to try to feel better can be an important step toward improvement. But while some people find that cultivating acceptance (Chapter 9) actually enhances their other SAD-fighting efforts right from the start of their SAD treatment, others will feel open to this new way of thinking only after they feel a little (or a lot) better. Throughout this book you will find reminders and tips for accepting SAD so you can move forward into the light.

> **How interested are you in building acceptance and reclaiming the joys of winter (on a scale of 1–10)?** _____
>
> **If you're interested in becoming more accepting of SAD and of winter, how do you think you might try to do that?**
>
> ☐ **Read Chapter 9.**
>
> ☐ **Remind yourself whenever you get down on yourself for being limited during your SAD season that having SAD is not your fault.**
>
> ☐ **Remember that you may not be able to eliminate all seasonal symptoms but you *can* gain big improvements with simple remedies.**
>
> ☐ **Think about the aspects of winter that can be enjoyable and how you can pursue them over time.**
>
> ☐ **Other:** _____

Stress Management (See Chapter 9)

For some people, unusual levels of stress during their low season can bring on SAD symptoms to a degree they don't typically experience. For others, stress just makes it harder to deal with the symptoms they usually do have. Either way, stress management is important to sailing through the winter. Because SAD hampers energy and concentration, it's a good idea to acknowledge that you're going to be less productive in the cold months. It's also wise to schedule those high-stress transitions and events—even the pleasant ones—for summer as much as is feasible. SAD stress management involves getting help where you can in the winter so you invest your energy where it's most critical. Some stressors, of course, can't be anticipated or can't be avoided even if you can see them coming. To reduce harmful inevitable stress, try meditation (Chapter 12). To minimize any guilt you feel about getting the help you need, cognitive-behavioral therapy (CBT; Chapter 14) can help you change unhelpful beliefs.

Pros

- Managing stress reduces cortisol levels and protects your overall health.

- Cutting back on winter commitments can allow you to use your creative energy where it matters most.

- Learning to manage your time realistically in the winter can improve your overall efficiency.

- Stress can often be managed via self-help.

Cons

- Overzealous stress management efforts (needing things to be 100% completed by winter, for example) can be stressful themselves.

- Minimizing commitments may mean risking disappointing others.

- Even though the methods are straightforward, stress is insidious, and you may need some help with pinpointing the best plan for you and sticking with it.

How interested are you in learning stress management methods (on a scale of 1–10)? _____

If you're interested in reducing and managing stress, how do you think you'd like to try to do it?

☐ Read Chapter 9.

☐ Try to cut down on obligations during your SAD season.

☐ Learn more about time management (online or by reading books on the subject).

☐ Explore meditation (Chapter 12).

☐ Try CBT methods to eliminate negative thoughts and pursue pleasant activities.

☐ Other: _____

Support

The support of others is almost always helpful for anyone struggling with a psychological problem like SAD. Depression has a way of draining us of the motivation and energy to stick to a course of action that can help, so encouragement, empathy, and a little nudge now and then can prove invaluable.

Pros

- Sharing experiences in support groups can provide ideas for improving SAD that you would not have thought of on your own.

- Support groups gather a wealth of resources, sparing you the task of researching sources of information and advice on your own.

- Support generally comes free of charge.

Cons

- Not everyone is comfortable sharing personal experiences, so trusting a close friend or relative who won't require that may be best.

- If revealing personal information to a group of strangers is uncomfortable for you, the cost of doing this may be higher in the form of stress than the return in the form of help or information.

- The only well-established support organization specifically for SAD is located in Great Britain, so access for those living elsewhere may be mainly online.

How interested are you in joining a support group or finding an individual who can support you in your efforts to deal with SAD (on a scale of 1–10)? _____

If you're interested in finding some support, how do you think you might go about it?

☐ Read Chapter 9.

☐ Identify confidants and go-to individuals who might offer a sympathetic ear and/or practical help.

☐ Figure out whether you can hire others to help with chores and routine tasks.

☐ Seek out a chat room or forum online.

☐ Try to find a support group.

☐ **Consider starting a local support group.**

☐ **Other:** _____

Meditation and Relaxation (See Chapter 12)

Meditation, a collection of ancient practices shown to improve depression, relieve stress, promote relaxation, and ease negative thoughts and cognitions, may help you fight SAD and generally improve your life. These methods need more study to examine whether they are specifically useful for SAD, but many of my patients have found them beneficial, and so have I. Another option that might help improve your mood and lower stress is progressive relaxation. Finally, there is a proven treatment for depression that combines mindfulness meditation with CBT, with powerful results.

Pros	**Cons**
• Meditation can be practiced easily at home on one's own.	• Many methods require instruction at first.
• Different forms of meditation seem to affect the brain in different ways, so if one type of meditation doesn't work for you, you can try others.	• It may take a few months before full results are felt.
• Meditation's effects often last beyond the period during which you're meditating, buffering you from stress and preparing you for your day.	• The best results come from daily meditation practice.
• Most practices require only 20 to 40 minutes per day.	
• Progressive relaxation is easy to learn.	

How interested are you in trying meditation practice or relaxation techniques (on a scale of 1–10)? _____

If you're interested in meditation or relaxation, how do you think you might pursue it?

☐ Read Chapter 12.

☐ Research transcendental meditation online.

☐ Attend a free transcendental meditation introductory session.

☐ Learn mindfulness meditation.

☐ Find progressive relaxation instructions online or in another book and learn them.

☐ Download or purchase recordings to assist with meditation or relaxation.

☐ Other: _____

Tapping the Success of CBT (See Chapters 13 and 14)

It's not hard to understand why we use words related to light to describe positive and negative thoughts and emotions. When you're in the middle of the winter, weighed down by SAD, your thoughts are dark, your mood black. And how do you behave under the pall of gloomy thoughts and feelings? Almost as if you're in mourning—immobilized, withdrawn, pessimistic, resigned. It's not your fault that you feel that way, but you may believe it is. In fact, you may harbor a whole host of negative beliefs about yourself and the world, and those beliefs in turn feed the symptoms of SAD and prevent you from fighting your way back to the light of day. You may also be subject to "wrong thinking," technically known as cognitive distortions, to unrealistic expectations, and other types of negative thinking that can destroy mood and color your actions.

It's a vicious cycle, to be sure. One way to disrupt the cycle is to use the powerful methods of CBT, a well-established treatment for depression that centers on the connection between what we think, what we feel, and what we do. CBT involves a variety of techniques and skills, specifically involving: (1) changing negative thoughts, (2) pursuing pleasant activities, and (3) engaging in psychotherapy with someone trained in this method.

Pros	Cons
• You can use basic CBT techniques by yourself.	• For full efficacy CBT requires commitment to practice.
• If you choose not to use light therapy or antidepressants, CBT alone may treat your SAD sufficiently.	• Without the quick boost that light therapy can provide, the mental focus and energy needed to use CBT methods may be more difficult.

- CBT seems to prevent relapses of SAD the next winter more effectively than light therapy given the previous winter.

- Some people need an experienced therapist to make the best use of CBT.

The *C* in CBT stands for "cognitive," which involves tackling negative thoughts to improve mood. The *B* for "behavioral" involves pursuing pleasant activities. Together, they can make future thinking more positive and encourage behavior that improves mood. Let's say you turn down a party invitation because you're experiencing SAD symptoms. You stay home and end up feeling lonely, isolated, and more down. But if you challenge the automatic negative thought—"I'll have a terrible time since I feel so lousy"—that comes after you receive the invitation, get dressed up, buy some flowers or a dessert to take to the party, and sally forth, more often than not you will end up feeling cheered by the company. You might even run into someone else with the winter blues and exchange your favorite remedies. You might end up feeling much better than you did before you got the invitation. That's how CBT works! Challenging negative thoughts and pursuing pleasant activities like social events can actually improve depression.

> *It can be tough to imagine all the activities and events that might be pleasant for you when you're depressed. To get an idea of what's available to you, do an Internet search for "pleasant activities list" or "pleasant events checklist." You'll be surprised by how many options you have.*

Because the methods of CBT are so concrete and standardized (often involving written homework), many people are quite successful doing it on their own. But many people do better with guidance and support. Some like the personal interaction and are more likely to stick with new efforts when they're accountable and have to show up somewhere on a schedule. If this sounds like you, psychotherapy might be a better choice than self-help alone. One limitation to professional help may be cost. If your insurance plan does not cover much of the expense, this may be a burden (and another burden is the last thing you need in the winter; see "Stress Management" later in this chapter). On the other hand, for someone who is unlikely to do CBT

> *If you need more help with CBT than what we could fit into this book, but you're not sure you have the resources to engage in psychotherapy, consider using Kelly Rohan's workbook* Coping with the Seasons, *which allows you to work through her anti-SAD program on your own, in detail.*

on his or her own and languishes in depression as a consequence, not getting help could be *more* costly.

> **How interested are you in learning CBT methods for changing negative thoughts (on a scale of 1–10)?**   _____
>
> **How interested are you in learning CBT methods for pursuing pleasant activities (on a scale of 1–10)?**   _____

Psychotherapy

When self-help CBT methods aren't enough, participating in psychotherapy with a professional might be beneficial. Other therapies may be useful as well, if you have problems that exist year-round and/or CBT doesn't seem to address them.

Pros	**Cons**
• For SAD complicated by other factors, professional help is likely to be more effective than self-help.	• Psychotherapy can be costly and may or may not be covered by your insurance plan.
• A therapist who comes to know you can help you work out new seasonal problems as they develop.	• Psychotherapy may be harmful if it does not improve depression or anxiety and discourages you from seeking medical treatment.
	• Therapists with expertise in SAD may be more difficult to find than those with expertise in depression in general.

> **How interested are you in learning CBT with a professional (on a scale of 1–10)?**   _____
>
> **How interested are you in learning CBT on your own (on a scale of 1–10)?**   _____
>
> **If you're interested in using CBT methods, how do you think you would use them?**
>
> ☐ **Read Chapters 13 and 14.**

☐ **Work on changing negative thoughts.**

☐ **Identify some pleasant activities that you'd enjoy and start scheduling them.**

☐ **Try CBT on your own.**

☐ **Seek professional help.**

☐ **Other:** _____

YOUR BRAIN CHEMISTRY

Like all depression, SAD has roots in the chemistry of your brain, but that chemistry is in turn influenced by your thoughts and behavior. Fortunately, there are many different routes by which you can influence your thoughts, behavior, *and* biochemistry to minimize or prevent seasonal symptoms.

Diet (See Chapter 11)

As you read earlier in the book, people with SAD often have carb cravings, perhaps due to a shortage of serotonin—a mood-enhancing neurochemical—in the brain. Where eating carbohydrate-rich foods seems to make others tired and lethargic, people with SAD tend to get a serotonin boost from carb consumption, which makes them feel more alert, albeit briefly. Managing your diet, especially in the winter, may have a significant effect on your seasonal depression, because overeating and being overweight are distressing. Although satisfying your carb cravings may make you feel temporarily better, the resulting weight gain with all of its health consequences makes it a self-defeating remedy.

Pros

- Healthy eating can restore some of the energy that SAD drains.

- Maintaining weight spares you the expense of buying larger clothes every winter.

- Avoiding gaining weight preserves self-esteem and prevents you from adding self-blame or shame to depression.

Cons

- Denying yourself the pleasure of eating whatever you crave can be tough when you're already feeling bad.

- Self-discipline requires mental focus you may lack during the winter and also tends to crack. (Antidote: a system of healthy rewards for good behavior!)

- Avoiding yo-yo dieting protects you from weight gain and the diseases it can lead to.

- To make the best food choices, you need to make yourself knowledgeable about nutrition.

- Sticking to good food choices requires some planning.

How interested are you in managing your diet to avoid seasonal weight gain and add energy (on a scale of 1–10)?   _____

If you're interested in changing your diet, what could you do?

☐ **Read Chapter 11.**

☐ **Plan your daily meals and snacks.**

☐ **Avoid buying carbohydrate-rich foods like cookies, candy, and chips.**

☐ **Buy some of the cookbooks listed in Chapter 11 to get new recipes.**

☐ **Consider cutting out excess caffeine and alcohol.**

☐ **Avoid marijuana and other substances.**

☐ **Other:** _____

Exercise (See Chapter 10)

You already know that where weight maintenance is concerned, diet and exercise together exert a more powerful effect than either one alone. Exercise can seem like a chore, but there are ways to make it work even in the midst of SAD.

Pros

- Exercise protects heart health and keeps weight under control.

- Aerobic exercise raises metabolic rate.

- Weight training builds muscle, and muscle cells have a higher metabolic rate than fat cells.

Cons

- It can be hard to muster the energy to get out of bed with SAD, let alone work out.

- It's hard to appreciate the mood and other benefits of exercise until you actually experience them.

- If you're pressed for time, you may feel like exercise is tough to schedule.

- Exercise can become a social event, adding to your daily pleasant activities.

- Outdoor exercise can increase your exposure to sunlight.

- Exercise boosts your sense of yourself as an active, vigorous person.

- Exercise may counteract weight gain from holiday eating.

- If you haven't been in the habit of regular exercise, you may need to do some reading, join a health club, or consult a personal trainer to determine the best program for you and how to get started.

- If you've been sedentary for a long time, you should consult your physician to get the go-ahead for the type of exercise you want to do.

How interested are you in exercising to maintain weight and boost health and mood (on a scale of 1–10)? _____

If you're interested in exercising, how could you plan to do it?

☐ **Read Chapter 10.**

☐ **Figure out what kind of exercise might feel like a pleasant activity rather than a chore.**

☐ **Find an exercise buddy.**

☐ **Identify ways to exercise outdoors to get extra sunlight.**

☐ **Join a gym.**

☐ **Hire a trainer.**

☐ **Sign up for calorie-burning, heart-bumping exercise classes.**

☐ **Other:** _____

Supplements (See Chapter 10)

Can vitamins, minerals, and herbs help? Possibly.

Pros

- Herbs and supplements don't require a prescription.

Cons

- The fact that you can buy supplements and herbs over the counter does not mean they are necessarily harmless.

- Fatty acids, available in fish oil supplements, may ease depression and are beneficial to the heart.

- Some supplements can be expensive.

- St. John's wort, an herbal antidepressant, photosensitizes users, meaning you risk sunburn or eye pain when taking it and exposed to sunlight or light therapy.

How interested are you in trying supplements (on a scale of 1–10)? _____

If you're interested in seeing whether supplements can improve your mood, how might you follow up on this interest?

☐ **Read Chapter 10.**

☐ **Try daily adding vitamins and omega-3 fatty acids.**

☐ **Experiment with St. John's wort if not using light therapy.**

☐ **Other:** _____

Negative Ions (See Chapter 8)

Positively charged ions in the air, like those that arrive with the Santa Ana winds in California, are widely considered by the general public to be bad for mental health. Does this mean that *negative* ions could have a beneficial effect on SAD? Apparently they do. (Remember: Even though the word "positive" is usually associated with well-being and the word "negative" with ill health, in this case it is the opposite.) A machine called a negative ion generator may duplicate the positive mood effects of standing near a waterfall or taking a walk on the seashore.

Pros

- Negative ions seem to have no side effects.

- You can purchase a reliable generator online.

Cons

- Only high-flow-rate generators produce dense enough negative ions to have any positive effect.

- The unit costs $100–200.

- Negative ion generators and light boxes cannot be used at the same time.

How interested are you in trying a negative ion generator (on a scale of 1–10)? _____

If you're interested in trying a negative ion generator, what steps would you like to take?

☐ Read Chapter 8.

☐ Buy a negative ion generator.

☐ Other: _____

Medication (See Chapter 15)

As noted earlier, I usually move on to medications when simpler measures, such as increasing light exposure and taking other self-help or psychotherapy measures, fall short. *But if you need more than light and stress management, medication can be more effective, more available, and less costly than even first-rate psychotherapy.* If your depression is resistant to other treatment efforts, there is every reason to consider the benefits that antidepressant medications can offer.

Pros

- When started before winter symptoms appear, antidepressants might prevent a SAD episode entirely.

- Most side effects are minor in most people.

- Bupropion, my first choice for people with SAD, has fewer side effects than other antidepressants (notably sexual difficulties, lethargy, and weight gain).

- Most first-choice antidepressants are available in generic form.

- You may be able to reduce the dosage or discontinue an antidepressant outside of winter.

Cons

- Full effects of antidepressants may take a few weeks to appear.

- Getting the medication and dosage right could take a few trials of several weeks each.

- All drugs can have side effects.

- Antidepressants require prescriptions, which involve psychiatrist/physician visits and drug purchases.

- Antidepressants should not be discontinued suddenly.

- Antidepressants may cause problems if taken during pregnancy.

How interested are you in trying an antidepressant (on a scale of 1–10)? _____

If you're interested in exploring medication, how would you follow through?

☐ Read Chapter 15.

☐ Talk to your physician about the possibility of trying medication.

☐ Try other remedies first, keeping medication in mind as another resource if simpler treatments don't provide enough improvement.

☐ Other: _____

WHICH TREATMENTS DO I WANT TO TRY FIRST?

Prepare

When doctors recommend treatments for any illness, they typically follow the guideline of starting with the simplest, least invasive option that seems likely to produce the greatest improvement. That's why I always start by recommending light therapy and suggesting basic modifications to the environment (more light and less stress). These methods are relatively easy to put in place, they can be used without professional help, they usually come with no side effects, and on the average they give a pretty good return for the investment. Next are methods for getting help and support (again, reducing stress), as well as learning acceptance of SAD and the limitations it imposes on you. As I said earlier, accepting that you'll still be left with some symptoms after putting in place your best SAD solution will take time. But starting out by recognizing SAD as a biological condition that you can't help having can ease the self-blame and guilt that only cause stress instead of easing it. You can also make lifestyle modifications on your own. While it may feel like a chore, diet and exercise are key to good mental and physical health in people with SAD. But do whatever you can to make these lifestyle changes rewarding. Chapters 10 and 11 will help in this regard—and so will Chapter 13, as you discover that some activities you find pleasant also get you moving, get you outdoors, and give you a mood-lifting alternative to the temporary boost of carb-rich foods. CBT offers straightforward methods for tackling automatic negative thoughts directly, and you can learn these on your own, although many people find it helpful to have the guidance and support of a therapist. Finally, there is medication. Although I don't tend to go for medications right off the bat, many of my patients find them invaluable.

There's a lot to consider when choosing which treatments to investigate. I've given you a basic path that I recommend to my patients, but beyond that a lot depends on your personal resources and preferences. Now that you've read the fundamentals of all your options, how do they stack up if you take into account the ratings you gave them above and your answers to the following questions?

Do you prefer to go it alone, or are you more comfortable working with an expert when you have a problem to address? _____

Is money a major consideration for you? _____

Are you interested in making changes that will require ongoing effort, with possibly additional benefits to your health and well-being outside of SAD, or do you prefer to "just take a pill" (literally or figuratively)? _____

Now look back at the ratings you gave to each treatment option above and list them in order from highest number to lowest:

Rating: _____ **Treatment:** _____

Rating: _____ **Treatment:** _____

Rating: _____ **Treatment:** _____

Rating: _____ **Treatment:** _____

Rating: _____ **Treatment:** _____

Rating: _____ **Treatment:** _____

Rating: _____ **Treatment:** _____

Rating: _____ **Treatment:** _____

Rating: _____ **Treatment:** _____

Rating: _____ **Treatment:** _____

Rating: _____ **Treatment:** _____

Rating: _____ **Treatment:** _____

Rating: _____ **Treatment:** _____

Rating: _____ **Treatment:** _____

Rating: _____ **Treatment:** _____

Rating: _____ **Treatment:** _____

Rating: _____ Treatment: _____

Rating: _____ Treatment: _____

Rating: _____ Treatment: _____

It's likely that some treatments received the same rating. No surprise there. It often helps to try more than one type of treatment at a time. If your SAD is very mild, however, you can try sequencing treatments one at a time, starting with the one that appeals to you most for all the reasons related to effectiveness, practicality, and personal lifestyle and resources:

The treatment I'd like to try first is: _____

At the same time, I'd like to try (if any):

_____

_____

If these approaches don't give me the relief I'm looking for, the next thing I'll do is:

_____

_____

If those don't work well enough either, I'll try this next:

_____

_____

Obviously, this is a preliminary plan, and you'll probably end up modifying it. Some treatments may prove more difficult to use than you anticipated. Some may surprise you with how easy they are to use and how beneficial.

In the next two chapters you can fill in this framework a little more, using planning tools that provide a simple, convenient way to sort out your thoughts and get a handle on SAD. If they don't seem likely to make your life easier, however, feel free to skip to Part II and get started on using the treatments, tools, and strategies that will make up your SAD Solution.

5

Planning to Beat SAD

Once you've identified the treatments you'd like to explore further, you need to know how to put them together into an effective treatment plan. If medication ends up as part of your plan, the prescribing physician can help you fit that into your overall regimen. If you're going to seek psychotherapy, your therapist can help you plan as well. But it's perfectly feasible to proceed with self-help, especially if your SAD is mild to moderate. You can start your planning by considering the same guidelines that I use in working with my patients.

Five Principles for Treating SAD

1. **Plan ahead.**

2. **Start treatment early.**

3. **Begin with the simplest treatment(s).**

4. **Add treatments in layers as needed.**

5. **Peel off the layers of treatment one by one as the days begin to lengthen again.**

1. PLAN AHEAD

Go back to page 29 and how you answered question 1 of the "How Seasonal Are You?" questionnaire. What month did you enter as the month you feel worst each year? _____

Now review how you answered items B–J for question 1:

If you're a **winter type,** write the months you entered for the following items here:

B _____

E _____

G _____

J _____

You probably chose December, January, or February for when you tend to gain the most weight (B), when you eat most (E), when you socialize least (G), and when you sleep most (J).

If you're a **summer type,** write the months you entered for the following items here:

D _____

F _____

G _____

I _____

You probably chose July or August for when you sleep least (D), lose most weight (F), socialize least (G), and eat least (I). Note that summer types often sleep and eat less (and lose weight) in the summer, when they're feeling their worst.

As discussed in Chapter 2, you could also have a summer–winter pattern. For the purposes of planning ahead there is a value to knowing when you are likely to start noticing symptoms and when you feel worst. You want to be prepared (the first P in your SAD Solution app) well before you feel your worst and ideally also before you notice symptoms, because that's when you'll have the most energy and focus for taking anti-SAD steps and because the earlier you take action, the greater the preventive effect (the second P in your SAD Solution APP).

From what you know now, when would you say your symptoms generally start?

_____

With that information alone, write down one thing you could do differently this year, before your symptoms begin (or, if they've already begun, next year before they begin):

_____

_____

_____

★ KEY POINTS

By the time you're feeling really SAD, it's later than it needs to be (although never too late!) . . . so try to plan and start treatment well before symptoms take hold.

Knowing Your Seasonality throughout the Year

Identifying your worst and best months is a good start on understanding your seasonal pattern, providing a basis for planning ahead. Symptoms of SAD often develop in a predictable sequence. Try numbering yours in the order in which you think they typically occur:

_____ Trouble waking up in the morning

_____ Reduced energy

_____ Carb cravings

_____ Increased appetite

_____ Weight gain

_____ Trouble concentrating

_____ Lowered sex drive

_____ Social withdrawal

_____ Depression, irritability, anxiety

Did you find it helpful to put your symptoms in order? Do you think it will act as an early warning system and a guide to planning? An interesting fact—one that many health care professionals don't realize—is that depression is typically a late symptom of SAD, and by its nature it tends to overwhelm other symptoms. Often,

SAD symptoms appear in roughly the order listed above. If that's true for you (even with a minor variation or two), you could plan ahead by knowing when you first start having difficulty getting out of bed in the morning. At this early point in your SAD, you probably still have the energy and focus most of the day to think about how you might head off the later symptoms. And it is often an excellent time to start implementing your SAD-busting routine (as detailed in Chapter 6). To get to know your SAD in detail, start monitoring your symptoms:

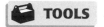 **TOOLS**

Tools You Can Use: A Journal or Calendar

Acquire a journal with a space to record changes in your thoughts, feelings, or physical activities—it can be a day planner type of book or an electronic application for your computer or smartphone. Plan to enter key points in your annual cycle, such as when specific symptoms appear and disappear, when your mood begins to dip, when it reaches its low point, when it begins to go back up and reaches its midline (when you're neither depressed nor elated), and when you feel elated or euphoric. Don't hesitate to enter any thoughts or emotions when you experience them. You can never tell what will prove most useful in your quest to beat SAD!

Here is an example showing some of the main points of interest for Diana's SAD:

> **Sept. 15:** Couldn't wake up this morning and missed my bus to work . . . felt groggy all day.

> **Sept. 18:** Even though it's Saturday and I slept in, I can't seem to focus on anything and am just sitting around watching TV.

> **Oct. 2:** Trying hard not to have a second doughnut for breakfast today . . . Can't wait for the day to be over so I can go home and just sit on the couch.

> **Oct. 29:** Canceled another date (the second this month) with Jeff. Just not interested.

> **Nov. 17:** Scale says I gained 3 pounds since last week . . . and Thanksgiving is next week!!!

> **Dec. 22:** Mom just called me for the *fifth* time this week about what we're going to serve at our Christmas Eve potluck. Ugh. I don't even want to see anyone. Need to force myself to go shopping this afternoon . . . 3-hour nap before dinner. Got nothing done. Just want to go back to bed.

> **Dec. 23:** *Can't* fit this shopping in!

Dec. 24: Feel my worst. Called Mom and started to cry. Now I feel like a big baby . . .

Jan. 15: Cruise is still 6 weeks away. Don't know how I'll make it till then . . .

Feb. 2: How am going to go on vacation when none of my summer clothes fit?

March 7: Back from the trip . . . instantly felt awful.

April 1: Joke's on me: I actually walked around this morning just to look at the crocuses poking up!

June 25: Took the whole day off. Couldn't concentrate on work and went running, then swimming. Then BBQ with friends. Great day!

Diana follows a familiar SAD pattern of starting to feel tired and groggy, sleeping too late, feeling hungry when she wouldn't be in the summer and early fall. By November she's getting irritable, and right before Christmas we can see she's irritated, frustrated, and has been having difficulty meeting obligations. Although you can't see it in the illustration, Diana didn't enter anything during the 2 weeks following Thanksgiving. She didn't have the energy and was ashamed of how she felt and how little she believed she was getting done—and by her weight, which continued to creep upward. *Note that not filling in a journal is perfectly okay—the last thing such tools should do is impose another obligation!* There's also a lot Diana can learn from what she has entered: The fact that her vacation was scheduled for the first week in March, which felt like an eternity away in mid-January might mean she should try scheduling it earlier next year. The fact that she reported feeling euphoric in June but couldn't get much done indicates she might have been feeling typical effects of hypomania—which might tell her that the big projects she wants to tackle should be scheduled for May, not the height of summer.

You don't need to wait until you've collected a lot of data to start thinking ahead. Fill out the form on the next page now and then review it next year to see if you want to change anything based on what you've learned about your relationship with the seasons.

2. START TREATMENT EARLY

With a good grasp of which symptoms you experience when, you can figure out when to start which treatments and nip many symptoms in the bud. This will give you a start on the month-by-month plan I'll help you draw up in Chapter 6.

Thinking Ahead:
How Can I Plan to Head Off SAD?

Make extra copies of this form so you can use it again as you learn more about your experience with SAD through the year. For now, though, write down any ideas you have about what you could accomplish in the summer, when energy is high (for winter SAD), to ensure that you're prepared. *It's okay for these to be just preliminary ideas. All the information you'll need to come up with concrete plans and follow through on them is in Part II.*

1. Do I need to see or line up any doctors or therapists?

    What to do: _____ When: _____

    What to do: _____ When: _____

    What to do: _____ When: _____

2. Do I need any equipment or supplies (light boxes, exercise equipment, etc.)?

    What to do: _____ When: _____

    What to do: _____ When: _____

    What to do: _____ When: _____

3. Do I need to devise any new plans (for diet, exercise, socializing, relaxation/meditation, etc.)?

    What to do: _____ When: _____

    What to do: _____ When: _____

    What to do: _____ When: _____

4. Should I plan for environmental changes (changing indoor light at home or work, booking a winter vacation, etc.)?

    What to do: _____ When: _____

    What to do: _____ When: _____

    What to do: _____ When: _____

For most people with winter SAD, the first symptoms are noticeable in September, meaning it would probably be a good idea to start some treatments by the beginning of that month or even earlier. For many people with SAD, late summer is a good time to have an annual physical. You can deal with any health problems that could complicate your seasonality early, and your physician can review with you how you've fared through the preceding year.

As the daily light begins to wane, it's a good idea to get as much natural light as you can, through outdoor exercise, recreation, landscaping/gardening, or even exterior house maintenance (see Chapter 10). To prevent morning grogginess from dawn arriving later and later, some people benefit from using a dawn simulator followed by regular light therapy (see Chapter 7). This may be the main treatment that you need, depending on how severe your seasonality is. If you need additional help, your doctor might prescribe medication and/or psychotherapy (see Chapters 14 and 15), and it's always a good idea to consider a winter vacation in a sunny, warm locale if it's feasible to take one (see Chapter 8).

This is just an example of how you might start your preventive and treatment efforts before SAD takes hold in a given year. Your own plan will be unique to you. At the end of Chapter 4 you formed a preliminary idea for what treatments you might start with. If you'd like to see how much further your understanding has come, add *when* you might want to start these treatments to the form on page 80. Don't feel like you have to fill out all six lines. Just enter any ideas you have at this point.

3. BEGIN WITH THE SIMPLEST TREATMENT

Prepare

What is simplest for you depends on your unique situation, although I consider increasing light comparatively simple for everyone. Beyond using a light box as explained in Chapter 7, did the pros and cons and fast facts in Chapter 4 help you get an idea of which treatments you found most appealing? We're all creatures of habit, and so what will be simplest for you to do next to get more light might be what's most familiar. If you've ever been an athlete, for example, it might be simple to drag out your outdoor sports equipment again, whereas if you've been sedentary, working out or playing a sport may seem like a complicated chore. If you're constantly weighed down by negative thoughts, you might appreciate using the thought-changing worksheets in Chapter 14. It's so much easier than trying to browbeat yourself into completing tasks, being sociable, or adopting healthy habits. Others may be so immobilized by low mood that medication may be the quickest and best solution. You can generally figure out what works best for you by trial and error. Remember, you know yourself best. When it comes time to devise your plan in Chapter 6, try to trust your own instincts and the understanding

When Should I Start Treating My SAD?

Treatment 1. _____ Starting on (date): _____

Treatment 2. _____ Starting on (date): _____

Treatment 3. _____ Starting on (date): _____

Treatment 4. _____ Starting on (date): _____

Treatment 5. _____ Starting on (date): _____

Treatment 6. _____ Starting on (date): _____

From *Winter Blues Survival Guide*. Copyright 2014 by The Guilford Press.

you are building—don't feel pressured to do what works for others you may know (or read about).

4. ADD TREATMENTS IN LAYERS AS NEEDED

Here's where awareness comes into play again. Keep in mind that the way you feel one day, or week, or month, is likely to change the next day, week, or month. That's the nature of seasonality. So you will want to recognize how your symptoms are changing and be ready to pull another prevention or treatment arrow out of your quiver as changes occur.

When you have SAD, you can feel like you're walking down a dark staircase as the days shorten, climbing back out of the basement only once the light shines down on you for longer periods every day. In fact, it's helpful to think of the course of SAD through the year as a staircase. The figure on the facing page shows how the symptoms of winter SAD typically worsen from September through January and don't usually begin to subside until February and March. The second bar graph in the figure shows how this corresponds with the length of the day during each

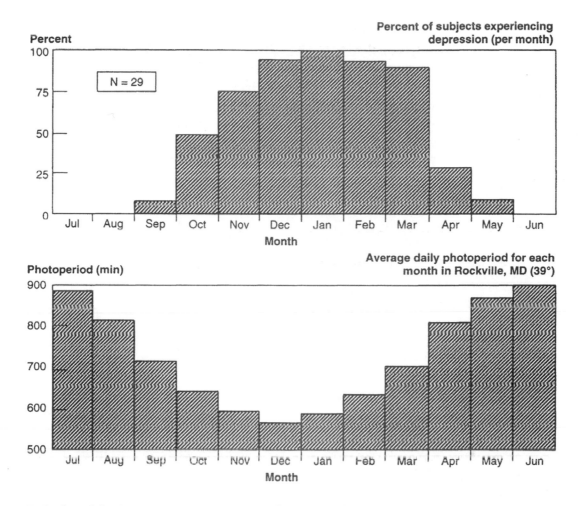

Relationship between symptoms of SAD and length of day. Reprinted from "Seasonal Affective Disorder: A Description of the Syndrome and Preliminary Findings with Light Therapy" by Norman E. Rosenthal et al., *Archives of General Psychiatry, 41*(1), 72–80 (1984). This figure is in the public domain.

month. Notably, there's a big leap up in symptoms in October even though the shift in day length isn't any greater, and there's a correspondingly precipitous drop in symptoms in April despite the fact that the days have been getting longer since the winter solstice. These observations may result from the *rate* of change in day length, which is greatest in late September and late March, at the time of the equinoxes. Our minds and bodies may pick up these rapid changes and respond accordingly. Or there may be certain thresholds in day length that, once crossed, trigger or relieve SAD symptoms.

Myth Buster: For most people with winter SAD, symptoms are still pretty severe in February and March, as shown in the figure on page 81. Shouldn't people be starting to feel relief, considering that the days are getting incrementally longer? It turns out that day length may not be the only relevant factor. The amount of light entering the eyes, at least in the East and Midwest, seems to be at its lowest after December—probably because the weather tends to be at its cloudiest. In the western United States this phenomenon might not be as common, but until the days get as long as they do in April or May, the rest of the northern United States may feel like it's draped in a shroud. In places where the ground is covered in snow, things can be better because snow reflects lots of light.

How Do You Know When to Add a Treatment Layer?

The first graph on page 81 shows how the severity of SAD tends to climb and then fall from autumn to spring. Monitoring severity is one way to plan ahead and know when to start treatments (see "Tools You Can Use" on page 85). But a good way to know when to boost treatment is to recognize when new symptoms appear. Let's say you start needing your alarm and the snooze button to get out of bed in mid-September; you could then take measures to add light to your bedroom earlier in the morning (see Chapter 8 for more about this). This may help a lot, so that you don't find yourself nodding off at your desk in late afternoon. But as September flows into October, you may find yourself heading for the vending machines in the afternoon and returning to your desk with candy bars or bags of chips. You start eating second helpings at dinner. These shifts in appetite are a new symptom that may signal it's time to add light therapy to your routine—and get serious about your diet. It's important to note these developments because if you start thinking that everything is just fine as long as you're not feeling outright depressed, you can end up walloped in midwinter without warning. Again, the staircase image is a good reflection of what might happen; page 83 shows the same symptoms that you numbered earlier, but the graphic image of steps may help keep you alert to what might come next as the days roll on.

☀ *Typical Steps of SAD Symptoms*

SAD often progresses in a stepwise fashion, adding symptoms in layers. Regard the early symptoms as a warning that you may feel depressed later. Whenever new symptoms appear—or old ones get worse—it may mean you're not using enough strategies and it may be time to consider adding another layer of treatment.

Sleeping more/having difficulty waking up

Waning energy

Carb cravings/increased appetite

Weight gain

Difficulty concentrating

Reduced sex drive

Socializing less/withdrawal from family and friends

Depression, irritability, anxiety

Note: you may want to amp up your current treatment regimen if you're not feeling better or are feeling worse. Although it's nice to be able to add treatments one at a time to know what's helping you most, in practice, especially if SAD symptoms are bad, it may be a better idea to pile on several treatments at the same time. Again, if you have already decided that light and other treatments, such as stress management efforts, would work equally well for you, trying to implement them at the same time is most likely to spare you the effects of insufficient treatment. Prevention is always better than playing catch-up.

Don't Change Your Regimen Too Quickly or Drastically

Prepare

Many treatments take time to produce their full effect or for the body and mind to adjust. One patient of mine with moderate SAD started light therapy for 15 minutes in the morning and evening once he started feeling the symptoms of SAD. His depression immediately lifted, but he also felt extremely jumpy, with a racing heart and headaches. I encouraged him to stick with light therapy but reduce its duration to 10 minutes in the morning only. Within 3 days the side effects stopped, but the mood benefit remained. Whatever treatment or treatments you are using, it is usually a good idea to hang in there for a couple of weeks *as long as side effects aren't severe or dangerous* so that you give the treatment a fair chance. If light treatment causes significant irritability, jumpiness, or racing thoughts, you should consult a doctor, as mania can be a significant problem.

5. PEEL OFF LAYERS OF TREATMENT ONE BY ONE AS THE DAYS LENGTHEN

Usually people know when they're feeling better and decrease their light and other remedies without too much difficulty—at least at first. But in spring the weather is changeable, and a patch of gray days can bring SAD symptoms right back again. So, as the days get sunnier, it's okay to peel back most treatments gradually. But keep your eyes on the skies and be ready to turn that light box on again. Consult with your doctor before changing medication dosages.

Although your pattern of symptoms can differ from year to year due to a number of variables, you can also anticipate when your symptoms might start to subside by looking at your history of symptoms from previous years. Think for a minute about your sleep habits as an example. If you sleep the most in January and the least in July, you're obviously starting to sleep normally somewhere in between. You can guess at when you start having less trouble waking up in the morning or having more energy in the afternoon. Or you can fill out the form that follows to look at how your sleeping habits vary from season to season and use this to plan for future years.

Circle the number of hours (including naps) that you sleep per day during each season.

Winter (Dec. 21–Mar. 20)	1 2 3 4 5 6 7 8 9 10 11 12 13 14 15 16 17 18 18+
Spring (Mar. 21–June 20)	1 2 3 4 5 6 7 8 9 10 11 12 13 14 15 16 17 18 18+
Summer (June 21–Sept. 20)	1 2 3 4 5 6 7 8 9 10 11 12 13 14 15 16 17 18 18+
Fall (Sept. 21–Dec. 20)	1 2 3 4 5 6 7 8 9 10 11 12 13 14 15 16 17 18 18+

Most people sleep longer in the winter than the summer. People in the northeastern United States sleep an average of 42 minutes more in the winter, and those with very mild seasonal symptoms sleep 1 hour and 42 minutes longer in winter. But those with SAD sleep 2.5 hours longer in winter. If that's true for you, you might think about whether it's time to start cutting back on treatments at the time when your night's sleep typically shortens and your daytime energy rises. What

TOOLS

Mood Ratings Chart

Scale: +50 = The best I've ever felt
0 = Even mood
-50 = The worst I've ever felt

Year	July	Aug.	Sept.	Oct.	Nov.	Dec.	Jan.	Feb.	Mar.	April	May	June
Last year												
2 years ago												
3 years ago												
4 years ago												
5 years ago												
Average												

symptoms you are experiencing at that time should be your primary guide, but knowing what you might expect throughout the year is an excellent planning tool.

Another way to get a good picture of when your symptoms begin, peak, subside, and then disappear entirely is to chart your mood over the years. Use the form on page 85 if you find it comforting to have a record to refer back to. If you can, think carefully about your experience over 5 years so that you can see where any pattern emerges.

🧰 TOOLS

Tools You Can Use: Your SAD Graph

If you prefer a visual picture to a bunch of numbers, you can take your average mood ratings and plot them on a line graph set up to represent the scale in your mood ratings table. Sometimes a visual curve sticks in the mind and can remind you through the winter of when you're likely to experience fewer SAD symptoms.

In general, however, when it comes to scaling back on treatments, how to proceed depends on whether you are working with a doctor or going it alone. It makes sense to involve your doctor in decisions about scaling back. It's almost never a good idea to stop medications abruptly, which is a setup for withdrawal symptoms, so be sure to consult your doctor before making changes in any medications you're taking.

If you're working on SAD on your own, scale back treatments gradually as the days lengthen. Usually this means reducing the duration of light therapy, whereas habits you've developed to combat SAD, like exercise and meditation, are likely to serve you well year-round. You might be surprised to know that some people continue light therapy (although much less of it) all year too. I am one of them. After a while, you'll develop a sense of when your light therapy is too little, too much, or just right.

A PRELIMINARY PLAN

If you feel like it will help you pull together what you've learned so far, use the form on pages 87–88 to jot down how you might apply the six treatment principles in this chapter. Remember, worksheets like this one are here for your benefit. Some people find them helpful; others don't. Use them if you are in the first group. Many people find their minds muddled and their memory faulty when they try to recon-

My Preliminary Plan for Beating SAD

What I will do to plan ahead (include dates):

_____

_____

_____

_____

When I will start treatment:

_____

Which treatment I will begin with:

_____

Which treatments I'll add:

When _____ happens (new symptom or severity
change), I will add _____ (new treatment), probably
around _____ (date)

When _____ happens (new symptom or severity
change), I will add _____ (new treatment), probably
around _____ (date)

When _____ happens (new symptom or severity
change), I will add _____ (new treatment), probably
around _____ (date)

When _____ happens (new symptom or severity
change), I will add _____ (new treatment), probably
around _____ (date)

When _____ happens (new symptom or severity
change), I will add _____ (new treatment), probably
around _____ (date)

When _____ happens (new symptom or severity
change), I will add _____ (new treatment), probably
around _____ (date)

My Preliminary Plan for Beating SAD *(cont.)*

How I'll stop treatments:

When _____ happens (symptom subsides or severity drops), I will cut back on or stop _____ (treatment), probably around _____ (date)

When _____ happens (symptom subsides or severity drops), I will cut back on or stop _____ (treatment), probably around _____ (date)

When _____ happens (symptom subsides or severity drops), I will cut back on or stop _____ (treatment), probably around _____ (date)

When _____ happens (symptom subsides or severity drops), I will cut back on or stop _____ (treatment), probably around _____ (date)

When _____ happens (symptom subsides or severity drops), I will cut back on or stop _____ (treatment), probably around _____ (date)

When _____ happens (symptom subsides or severity drops), I will cut back on or stop _____ (treatment), probably around _____ (date)

struct their experiences from years past. Keeping notes can be comforting and helpful. If you prefer, feel free to proceed to Chapter 6 and use the planning form provided there.

You might take the same approach to filling out these forms as I suggested earlier regarding social activities or exercise. Make a little bit more effort than you really want to and see if you get benefits that repay your investment. Arriving at your SAD solution is always a matter of trying new things a bit at a time, seeing how your experience affects your thinking, and using what you learn to gather up all those small wins into a much bigger victory over SAD.

6

Tailoring Your Plan

Awareness, Preparation, and Prevention throughout the Revolving Year

As valuable as it is to understand what happens at the time of year when SAD begins, it's also helpful to know when you start to emerge from depression and what the other seasons are like for you. The Mood Ratings Table and SAD Graph in Chapter 5 can give you a clear picture of how you tend to feel throughout the year. If you're a record-keeping enthusiast, you can go back to these tools, any journal you're keeping, or even your Daily Mood Log and get a more specific view of how you feel month to month. If your memory seems vague on these shifts, you might want to peruse what you've recorded so far. Otherwise, just jot down some simple notes about your tendencies over the last few years in the form on page 90.

PLANNING MONTH BY MONTH

Stress management, which is such an important part of your SAD solution, is largely about what's going on around you and how you're expected (by yourself and others) to participate. It's also about taking advantage of your highest-energy periods to get things done that will spare you exhaustion and guilt during your lowest-energy times. In the following pages you'll find prompts to help you anticipate what usu-

My SAD Month to Month

Month	Mood (1 = lowest → 10 = highest)	Other issues: energy, pain, etc.
January		
February		
March		
April		
May		
June		
July		
August		
September		
October		
November		
December		

From *Winter Blues Survival Guide*. Copyright 2014 by The Guilford Press.

ally happens during each season and how you can use that information to plan to be good to yourself—especially when you need it most.

Remember, your SAD Solution APP starts with awareness, which fuels the preparations that lead to prevention.

SAD Solution APP

Be Aware   Prepare   Prevent

Summer: June, July, and August

What events typically occur in your life every summer or will occur this summer?

June:

Kids out of school for summer vacation? _____

College kids return home for summer? _____

School year ends for you (if you're a student or teacher)? _____

Graduations? _____

Summer vacation trip? _____

Visits to or from family? _____

Relocation to a summer home (all summer or every weekend)? _____

Weddings, birthdays, anniversaries, holidays? _____

Work projects/deadlines? _____

Physical problems brought on by the season (allergies, arthritis flare-ups, fibro-myalgia, etc.)? _____

_____

Anniversaries of sad events? _____

Other? _____

_____

July:

Kids leave for summer camp? _____

Family reunion? _____

Weddings, birthdays, anniversaries, holidays? _____

Vacation trip? _____

Work projects/deadlines? _____

Physical problems brought on by the season (allergies, arthritis flare-ups, fibro-myalgia, etc.)? _____

Anniversaries of sad events? _____

Other? _____

_____

August:

Kids return from camp? _____

Getting ready for school? _____

Kids going off to college? _____

Returning from summer home? _____

Weddings, birthdays, anniversaries, holidays? _____

Work projects/deadlines? _____

Physical problems brought on by the season (allergies, arthritis flare-ups, fibro-myalgia, etc.)? _____

_____

Anniversaries of sad events? _____

Other? _____

_____

The goal is to *anticipate* events that might cause you problems related to SAD. For example, many people find that, despite feeling at their peak during summer, they feel almost too good to get their best work done, especially creative work. Euphoria takes hold and distracts them from putting nose to grindstone to get things done. The lesson here might be that summer may not be the ideal time to plan on doing something like writing a book, especially if you think you might end up having to finish up in fall, when SAD is starting to bring you down. Individuals differ, however. While some people with SAD feel scattered during the summer, I find summer a particularly productive time. Therefore we need to know ourselves to plan effectively.

Think of other major commitments that would strain ordinary people—becoming chairperson of a committee, taking responsibility for a newsletter, taking on the running of a food pantry—anything requiring effort and time with deadlines attached. Summer is the time when you probably pack your days with enjoyable activities that are too hard to do during winter. Take advantage of your energy and enjoy every event that you can. Allowing a little time for planning for winter will pay off enormously and barely cut into the time you want to—and have a right to—devote to living a full and happy life.

How do you think predictable events for the summer might affect your seasonality, both during the summer and how you plan for fall and winter?

_____

_____

_____

How could you prepare for SAD during summer?

☐ Take shorter vacations (or no vacation) during summer so you can use your vacation time for a winter getaway to a sunnier clime?

☐ Plan stressful events (family reunions, other celebrations) usually scheduled in winter for summer instead, where feasible?

☐ Schedule big projects (moving, remodeling, etc.) for summer instead of winter, especially where you can be sure they will be completed well before your SAD symptoms kick in?

☐ Plan for the winter (everything from stocking up where practical to limit winter shopping to scheduling doctor's appointments and making environmental changes you'll appreciate in winter, like repainting walls or relighting rooms)? (Refer back to Chapter 5, where you entered some ideas for planning ahead, if you like, but always keep this thought in mind: It's important to have fun in summer!)

☐ Other? _____

_____

September: The First of Fall

What events occur in your life every September or will occur this September?

Back to school/college (the kids and/or you)? _____

Weddings, birthdays, anniversaries, holidays? _____

Work projects/deadlines? _____

Vacations? _____

Fall cleaning or autumn home repairs? _____

Physical problems brought on by the season (allergies, arthritis flare-ups, fibromyalgia, etc.)? _____

_____

Anniversaries of sad events? _____

Other? _____

_____

September might still feel like summer all month long, depending on where you live and how severe your winter blues are, but the days definitely are getting shorter in the northern hemisphere. So this is a good time to be alert for the first subtle shifts toward SAD. If summer is your favorite time of year, you might feel a little blue just because there's no denying that your days of beach weather are numbered, even if your symptoms haven't begun. And there are reminders everywhere, like autumn leaves and fall catalogs.

Even though the days may be sunny in September, some people are already feeling definite signs of SAD and should swing into full blues-beating mode. If the form at the beginning of the chapter revealed a dip in your mood in September, this definitely applies to you.

Prevent **How do you think predictable events for September might affect your seasonality, both now and later in the fall and winter?**

_____

_____

_____

How could you prepare for SAD during September? (Refer back to Chapter 5, where you recorded ideas for planning ahead, if you like.)

☐ Have your annual physical and also see your therapist, dietician, or other professionals who can help you prepare for winter?

☐ Purchase or replace light fixtures or light tubes?

☐ Get ahead on projects you couldn't reschedule for summer so that they don't all fall during winter?

☐ Do holiday preparation now instead of in November and December?

☐ Start stocking your freezer with soups and other comfort foods—chili, stews, casseroles—that aren't packed with starches and sweets but will appeal to you in winter?

☐ Spend as much time outdoors, in the sunlight, as you can?

☐ Start looking at possibilities for winter vacations?

☐ Review your diet and exercise regimens and make shifts toward health now?

☐ Catch up with friends and family now, before you feel less sociable?

☐ Keep windows unobstructed when you go to bed so the first rays of dawn sunlight reach your bed?

☐ Start using a dawn simulator?

☐ Other? _____

_____

October: Autumn's Peak

What events occur in your life every October or will occur this October?

Turning the heat on and closing the windows? _____

Weddings, birthdays, anniversaries, holidays? _____

Work projects/deadlines? _____

Vacations? _____

Yard cleanup and storage of outdoor furniture? _____

Shifts in available fresh foods and cooking styles? _____

Physical problems brought on by the season (allergies, arthritis flare-ups, fibromyalgia, etc.)? _____

Anniversaries of sad events? _____

Other? _____

_____

It's harvest time in the North, which is a time to celebrate the bounty summer has produced. Celebrate the harvest as much as you can, and remember that even if the farmers' markets are ending, there are fresh fruits and flowers available year-round (even if they are more expensive). Post-autumn equinox, the days are really getting shorter, and when the sun goes down, so does the temperature. Halloween and Day of the Dead are ways to celebrate the darker phases of the annual cycle. As of 2012, daylight savings time extends to the beginning of November, which means that the mornings can be dark until many people are preparing for, or on their way to, work and school.

🔆 *Be Sure to Prepare for Anniversaries of Sad Events*

If a sad event occurred during one of your SAD months in the past, that time of year is probably doubly hard for you. Some people mistakenly attribute reexperiencing this sadness to SAD, and others attribute their seasonal symptoms to their painful memories. The effects of the anniversary will pass, but during this period of time it's best to take extra care of yourself:

- Ask those close to you to give you extra support at this time.

- Cut yourself some slack and plan fewer obligations at this time.

- Find some small way to come to terms with the anniversary, such as visiting a place that reminds you of a lost loved one or making a donation (as affordable) to a charitable organization related to your loss.

Here is where a bit of mindfulness, described in Chapter 12, can help. Allow yourself to feel the sad feelings and watch them as they come . . . and go, knowing that they are all part of our ever-changing world, just like the seasons.

How do you think predictable events for October might affect your seasonality, both now and later in the fall and winter?

_____

_____

_____

How could you prepare for and deal with SAD during October? (Refer back to Chapter 5, where you recorded ideas for planning ahead, if you like.)

☐ Start using your light box as described in Chapter 7, perhaps 15 minutes in morning and evening. Use your awareness of your own internal state as your guide to whether, and how much, light therapy to start using; check your journal to see whether you notice a decline.

☐ Get up later in the morning, if feasible, so that you're not forced to get going in the dark.

☐ Find ways to celebrate the fall colors: apple picking, a trip to a pumpkin farm, football games at bright outdoor stadiums, hikes in the midday sun. Planning pleasant events (Chapter 13) is hugely helpful for anyone with SAD.

☐ Be sure your dawn simulator (Chapter 7) is set to account for the longer darkness in the morning.

☐ Buy some brightly colored sweaters, scarves, warm socks—anything that will help you associate cold weather with brightness instead of darkness.

☐ Celebrate the harvest by preserving foods and stocking up for the winter.

☐ Continue advance holiday preparations.

☐ Throw a simple Halloween party. (If your symptoms haven't started in ear nest, this can be a good annual tradition for socializing before you don't feel up to it. Think of socializing as a pleasant event with a hidden bonus— you not only get out and do something fun but usually get the support and friendship of others.)

November: No More Daylight Savings Time

What events occur in your life every November or will occur this November?

Weddings, birthdays, anniversaries, holidays? _____

Work projects/deadlines? _____

Vacations? _____

Replacing lighter-weight clothing in your closets with winter clothes? _____

Physical problems brought on by the season (allergies, arthritis flare-ups, fibromyalgia, etc.)? _____

_____

Anniversaries of sad events? _____

Other? _____

_____

The first weekend in November is the time that (as of 2012) the United States turns back its clocks an hour, ending daylight savings time. For many people, the extra daylight in the morning doesn't compensate for dusk that falls as early as 4:30 P.M. There's a distinct chill in the air up north, and some places will even see their first snows of the season. Thanksgiving can be a mixed blessing—fun if it doesn't cause you too much stress; a burden if being a gracious host or a grateful guest takes too much out of you.

How do you think predictable events for November might affect your seasonality, both now and later in the fall and winter?

_____

_____

_____

How could you prepare for and deal with SAD during November? (Refer back to Chapter 5, where you recorded ideas for planning ahead, if you like.)

☐ Up your light therapy to 30–45 minutes in morning and evening.

☐ Consider especially increasing the duration of evening light therapy to counteract the extra hour of darkness at the end of the day.

☐ Start routinely taking morning walks or bike rides (or other outdoor exercise) now that it's lighter in the mornings.

☐ Make every effort to stick to whatever exercise routine you've established so that you don't have to dredge up the impetus to start all over in winter.

☐ Plan to start taking medication if this has been part of your treatment (see Chapter 15), or talk to your doctor about whether you should start a trial of antidepressants this year.

-☀- ***Don't just start taking last year's unfinished prescription!***

Even if you know you usually start an antidepressant in November (or any other time of year), always check with your doctor before taking any pills left over from last year or before refilling a prescription that's still current.

☐ Ask everyone to bring a dish for Thanksgiving if you usually host, or suggest a change this year to having dinner at someone else's home. (Or order a catered dinner if feasible.) The holidays represent a challenge for most people with SAD, but they *can* be managed. See December, below, and also Chapter 9, which offers lots of ideas for managing time, accepting your limitations, and getting support from others during the holidays to prevent them from being a source of stress—without robbing yourself of their joys and comfort.

December: The Darkest Days and the Brightest Lights

What events occur in your life every December or will occur this December?

Dealing with snow? _____

Weddings, birthdays, anniversaries? _____

Celebrations of Christmas, Hanukkah, New Year's Eve? _____

Work projects/deadlines? _____

Vacations? _____

Participating in winter sports? _____

Physical problems brought on by the season (allergies, arthritis flare-ups, fibromyalgia, etc.)? _____

_____

Anniversaries of sad events? _____

Other? _____

_____

December and its festivities are a mixed blessing for those with SAD. The bright lights, blazing fires, and holiday cheer can elevate the spirits, and that's exactly what they were meant to do, to counteract the darkness of the season. But this is a time of year when acceptance of your limitations can be in short supply since the holidays also seem to require lots of work for everyone. The best approach, especially if you find yourself feeling ashamed of being unable to cope, is to ask yourself "How can I make the holidays work for *me*?" Trade-offs may be necessary, but they don't have to mean you miss out on the fun just to make the holidays enjoyable for others. See Chapter 9 for ideas, and when you're making sure you insert pleasant activities into your days as discussed in Chapter 13, be sure to come up with specific, *simple* ones for the holidays: A cup of cocoa with the kids? Taking photos of the family building a snowman? A favorite holiday movie on TV?

> **How do you think predictable events for December might affect your seasonality, both now and later in the winter?**
>
> _____
>
> _____
>
> _____

> **How could you prepare for and deal with SAD during December? (Refer back to Chapter 5, where you recorded ideas for planning ahead, if you like.)**

☐ Take advantage of all the light-centered traditions of the holidays, from decorating with Christmas lights, to lighting the menorah during Hanukkah, to keeping a fire going in your fireplace.

☐ Ask for help (or pay for it if affordable) with decorating and preparing for the holidays to make sure you don't miss the opportunity but do skip the stress. See Chapter 9 for help with becoming comfortable enough with SAD to ask, and get creative about how to make this work for you, including offering to reciprocate during summer.

☐ Ask for the understanding of family and friends regarding your need to limit your activities even though you'd love to celebrate too.

☐ Offer to host a spring, summer, or even fall holiday (depending on your seasonal pattern) in exchange for not hosting a winter holiday.

☐ Increase your light therapy as needed.

☐ Work hard at not feeling guilty about your limitations. (See Chapter 9 for help with acceptance and Chapter 14 for help with changing negative thinking.)

☐ *Take along your light fixture and/or dawn simulator if you travel over the holidays.*

☀ *Is Your SAD Compounded by the Holiday Blues?*

Although the phenomenon of depression specifically during the holidays has been hard to document scientifically, there seems little doubt that some people do view the holidays with dread and sorrow. Especially if you inherited SAD from a parent, your memories of the holidays may be colored by your disappointing experience of childhood celebrations. If you feel like your mood gets worse during the holidays, talk to someone about it—perhaps even a therapist—and get the help you need. It helps to gain an understanding of why you feel the way you do, and it will certainly help to get treatment to ease your depression.

Midwinter: January and February

What events occur in your life every winter after the holidays or will occur this winter?

January:

Dealing with snow? _____

Weddings, birthdays, anniversaries? _____ _____

Post-holiday blues? _____ _____   _____   _____

Work projects/deadlines? _____

Vacations? _____

Participating in winter sports? _____

Physical problems brought on by the season (allergies, arthritis flare-ups, fibromyalgia, etc.)? _____

_____

Anniversaries of sad events? _____ _____

Other? _____

_____

One of the most significant problems for many people in January is the letdown that follows the holidays. If the holidays are typically a trial for you, you may not feel the post-holiday blues on top of SAD, but the prospect of a few more months of short days can be tough to take. This is when it's particularly important to have pleasant activities (see Chapter 13) lined up, and if you have managed to schedule a vacation in the sun (Chapter 8), do what you can to look forward to it: look at brochures or websites of your destination, do a little shopping for resort wear online, tack up posters of your destination as happy reminders.

February:

Dealing with snow? _____

Weddings, birthdays, anniversaries? _____

Work projects/deadlines? _____

Vacations? _____

Participating in winter sports? _____

Physical problems brought on by the season (allergies, arthritis flare-ups, fibromyalgia, etc.)? _____

_____

Anniversaries of sad events? _____

Other? _____

_____

For many people—with and without SAD—February can seem like the darkest month of the year. Holiday cheer is a distant memory, and another couple of months of winter lie ahead. As mentioned earlier in the book, this time of year also seems to be particularly cloudy in much of the North. Again, a vacation south can be the best antidote. If not, preparing to get through this month as well as you can is more important than at any other time of year. Keep stress at a minimum (Chapter 9), treat yourself to enjoyable moments throughout the day (Chapter 13), take advantage of the stress-defusing effects of meditation and relaxation (Chapter 12).

How do you think predictable events for January and February might affect your seasonality, both now and later in the winter?

_____

_____

_____

How could you prepare for and deal with SAD during January and February? (Refer back to Chapter 5, where you recorded ideas for planning ahead, if you like.)

☐ Seek the light relentlessly. Get outside in the sun, especially when there's snow to reflect the sunlight, or if it's too cold, take a drive. Spend indoor time in the brightest room you have access to. Use your dawn simulator and light box every day.

☐ Cut back on chores and other drudgery and replace them with scheduled pleasant events.

☐ Increase or at least maintain your exercise routine.

☐ Consider medications if winter is getting to you without them (or talk to your doctor about changing your medications if they're not sufficient).

☐ Buy new houseplants (or forced bulbs, which will remind you that spring is around the corner when they bloom).

☐ Practice acceptance of winter and of the need to hibernate.

☐ Meditate or use positive imagery of springtime, which always arrives.

Spring: March, April, and May

What events occur in your life in the spring or will occur this spring?

March:

Weather changes? _____

Weddings, birthdays, anniversaries? _____ _____

Holidays? _____ _____

Work projects/deadlines? _____ _____

Vacations? _____ _____

Physical problems brought on by the season (allergies, arthritis flare-ups, fibromyalgia, etc.)? _____ _____

Anniversaries of sad events? _____ _____

Other? _____ _____ _____

_____

March is a transitional month. Depending on where you live, it might really feel like spring has sprung, or it might feel like winter is hanging on. Or you might feel as if you're bouncing between winter and spring during a single day in March (or April). Because this time of year is such a tease, I call it No Man's Land and always have to remind myself to keep up my light therapy, because spring is not yet here to stay. For most people with SAD, March remains a symptom-filled month.

April:

Weather changes? _____

Weddings, birthdays, anniversaries? _____

Holidays? _____

Work projects/deadlines? _____

Spring cleaning? _____

Vacations? _____

Physical problems brought on by the season (allergies, arthritis flare-ups, fibromyalgia, etc.)? _____

Anniversaries of sad events? _____

Other? _____

_____

Again, depending on where you live, April may bring full-blown spring, just a few crocuses peeking out of the snow, or the cold and damp of the legendary April showers. You might start to feel exhilarated, with your symptoms plummeting, or strangely irritated as you wrestle with volatile weather and an impatience to see the last vestiges of winter disappear.

May:

Weather changes? _____

Weddings, birthdays, anniversaries? _____

Holidays? _____

Work projects/deadlines? _____

Vacations? _____

Planning for the end of the school year? _____

Graduations? _____

Planting gardens and the beginning of yard work? _____

Getting a summer home ready for the season? _____

Physical problems brought on by the season (allergies, arthritis flare-ups, fibromyalgia, etc.)? _____ _____

Anniversaries of sad events? _____

Other? _____

_____

In most of the northern United States and Europe, spring has finally arrived
sometime in May. Flowers are everywhere, the sun's warmth can be felt on faces,
and everyone suddenly seems to be outdoors. For people with SAD, this is generally a prime month for both mood and productivity. In fact, if you have wintertime
SAD, May might seem uneventful since you probably have few reminders that you
are vulnerable to the change of seasons. The height of summer is still far off, and
all seems right with the world.

How do you think predictable events for spring might affect your seasonality?

_____

_____

_____

**How could you prepare for and deal with SAD during spring? (Refer back to
Chapter 5, where you recorded ideas for planning ahead, if you like.)**

☐ Recognize that this is a transitional time and stay aware of the changing
weather, which might vault you into summer euphoria but then yank you
back into the winter doldrums.

☐ Keep using light therapy as needed, gradually tapering it off once spring
seems here to stay.

☐ Participate in spring rituals to celebrate the return of your best time of year
(opening day of baseball season, May Day, a Memorial Day weekend trip
to a pretty spot).

☐ Catch up on chores you (wisely) put off in winter.

☐ Reward yourself for getting through another winter.

☐ Take advantage of this productive time and start your creative projects now.

☐ Schedule least-enjoyed tasks for now, when they're likely to impose minimal stress—and to free yourself up for the bacchanal of summer.

CREATING AN ANNUAL PLAN FOR BEATING SAD

Now you have everything you need to put together a plan for what you will do to beat SAD during every month of the year. Your plan should include ways to get optimal light, measures to ease stress and modify negative thinking, and methods for influencing biochemistry to minimize SAD symptoms—everything from diet and exercise to meditation and medication. Your plan should focus on awareness, preparation, and prevention (your SAD Solution APP), which means it should include steps for planning ahead throughout the year, taking advantage of the best of times and insulating yourself against the worst. Don't forget to include specific types of pleasant events you could pursue in each month of the year and how you might socialize, both to lift your spirits through laughter and to elicit needed support.

Make multiple copies of the blank form on pages 107–110 or download it from *www.guilford.com/rosenthal3-forms* so that you can revise it as needed, based on what you learn by monitoring your seasonality throughout the coming year. The form includes a space to record the action you plan to take, the date you will take it, and whether you have followed through on that aspect of the plan. If the data you've gathered in the preceding chapters is fresh in your mind, go ahead and start filling out the form. If you like, flip back through the preceding chapters to see if you omitted anything important that you entered in the worksheets.

To help you determine when you need to revise your plan, you already have tools like a journal and/or the Daily Mood Log on page 111. But each chapter in Part II ends with spaces to enter any changes you might decide to make based on what you've learned from reading about each treatment and from your experiences once you try the treatment. If record keeping seems like too much "homework," try to remind yourself that every trend it reveals to you can add one more small win to your SAD solution: Does skipping light therapy for a couple of days affect you on those days or for a few days later as well? Do your symptoms seem to vary depending on the time of the month (because the season is changing, because there's a holiday or other event at some point, or because of your menstrual cycle)? Looking at what you've recorded, what would you do differently next month or during this month next year?

My Annual Plan for Beating SAD

If an action entered in the form below will be taken throughout the month, versus on a particular starting date, on one day only, or on a range of dates, insert "ALL." Check off each action as it is completed (or started). You may need more space for action items, in which case download the form from *www.guilford.com/rosenthal3-forms* and modify it by adding more spaces as needed. Filling out the form on your computer would also allow you to store and easily revise your plan if you don't want to use a printed version.

Date	Action	✓
	January	
	February	
	March	

(cont.)

My Annual Plan for Beating SAD *(cont.)*

Date	Action	✓
	April	
	May	
	June	
	July	

My Annual Plan for Beating SAD (*cont.*)

Date	Action	✓
	August	
	September	
	October	
	November	

(cont.)

My Annual Plan for Beating SAD *(cont.)*

Date	Action	✓
	December	

In Part II of this book you'll find practical information and advice that will help you make the most of each treatment that has helped those with SAD reduce the impact of seasonality, cope with symptoms, and even prevent episodes. You now have an idea of which treatments you want to start with or focus on. Your SAD solution awaits you in Chapters 7–15. So let's get started!

SAD Solution APP-T

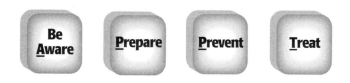

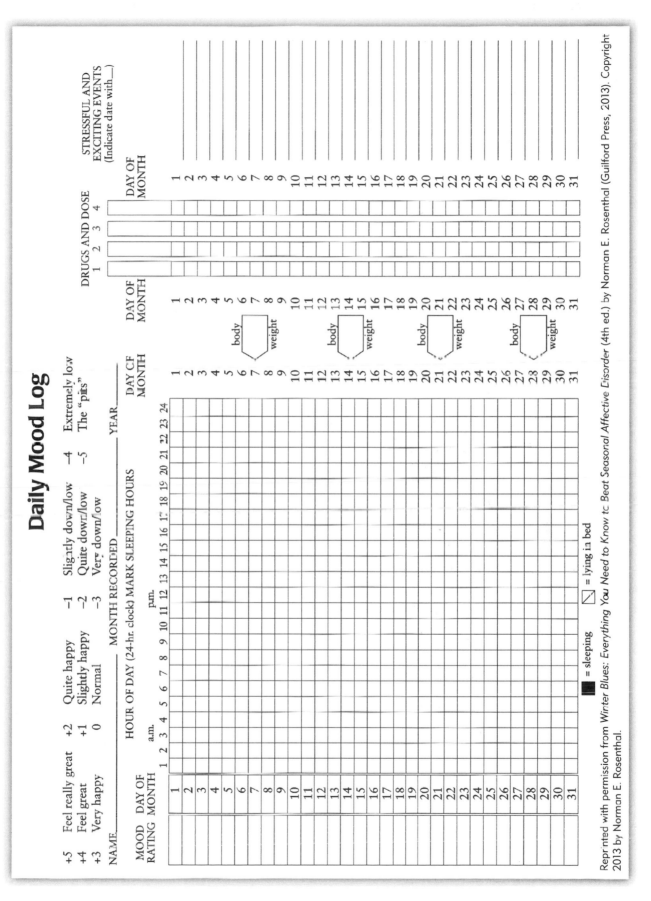

Daily Mood Log

+5	Feel really great	+2	Quite happy	−1	Slightly down/low	−4	Extremely low
+4	Feel great	+1	Slightly happy	−2	Quite down/low	−5	The "pits"
+3	Very happy	0	Normal	−3	Very down/low		

NAME _____   MONTH RECORDED _____ YEAR _____

■ = sleeping   ◰ = lying in bed

Reprinted with permission from *Winter Blues: Everything You Need to Know to Beat Seasonal Affective Disorder* (4th ed.) by Norman E. Rosenthal (Guilford Press, 2013). Copyright 2013 by Norman E. Rosenthal.

Part II

Treatments, Tools, and Strategies You Can Use

Light Therapy

Light is your first and best friend, whether you're just starting to address your SAD or trying to improve a treatment regimen you already have in place.

This chapter explains what you need to know to prepare for light therapy, to get started, to get the greatest possible benefit, to monitor your reaction, and to troubleshoot any problems you encounter.

↗ FAST FACTS

- Light therapy has been found helpful for 60–80% of people with SAD.
- A self-help trial of light therapy should last only 2 weeks. If it doesn't help, consult a professional.
- Light fixtures should be returnable for a full refund within 30 days of purchase.
- Light therapy is best started at the first signs of SAD, which may occur as early as August.
- There is no evidence that light therapy *properly administered* is harmful to the eyes.
- Light therapy is safe during pregnancy.
- Your insurance company might cover the cost of a light fixture.

- Dawn simulators work during sleep because the eyes are particularly sensitive to light before dawn.

- Dawn simulators may be especially useful for those who frequently travel to different time zones.

- A timer attached to a bedside lamp can substitute well for a dawn simulator even though the light goes on abruptly instead of gradually.

WHAT DO YOU HOPE TO GET OUT OF LIGHT THERAPY?

☐ I'm hoping it will be the only treatment I'll need to manage my SAD symptoms.

☐ I hope it will be a big part of my treatment but expect to need other help too.

☐ I've been trying other treatments for depression generally and would like to add light therapy now that I know I have seasonal symptoms.

☐ I have mild SAD and hope that light therapy will bump up my mood and productivity during my typical winter slump.

☐ I have few or no expectations but feel like I have little to lose by trying it.

WHERE DOES LIGHT THERAPY FIT INTO YOUR TREATMENT PLAN?

It will be the _____ (first, second, third, etc.) treatment I try in My Annual Plan for Beating SAD (Chapter 6).

I will plan to begin using light therapy around _____ (date) but will start earlier (or later) according to when my symptoms appear.

I plan to use _____ (type of light fixture).

I will try _____ minutes of light therapy at _____ (time of day) every day.

PREPARING FOR LIGHT THERAPY

TOOLS

A Light Box or a Pill Box?

If you're wondering whether you should just skip trying out light therapy and get a prescription for an antidepressant, know that two studies of Prozac versus light therapy showed the two to be just about equal in their benefits for those with SAD. However, there are several reasons *not* to skip light therapy and go straight to medication:

- Medication can have unpleasant side effects, such as increased weight and decreased interest in sex. Neither of these is a side effect of light therapy.

- Light therapy takes effect faster.

- Light therapy may be less expensive. Your insurance plan might not cover antidepressants fully or may not cover one that is "nonformulary" (not included on the insurance plan's list of preferred drugs) or not available in generic form. If a light box you buy doesn't meet your expectations, you can return it within the time period stated by the seller (usually 30 days).

You may have already figured out in Part I of this book what treatment appeals to you most to try first, and you can go back to Chapter 4 to review the pros and cons of light therapy and medication if you like.

Desirable Light Box Features

- Fluorescent (first choice) light bulbs

- Emission of 2,500 to 10,000 lux (the higher the better)

- Plastic diffuser to spread light

- UV filter to block rays coming from fluorescent bulbs

- A money-back return policy that gives you at least 30 days to try out the fixture

- Larger size (at least 1 foot square)

⚗ SCIENCE

The Science Scoop on the Best Light Box Features

- *Fluorescent bulbs are best.* These bulbs spread out the light maximally, while incandescent bulbs emit intense light from a small source, which could endanger your eyes if stared at directly. LED lights (white and blue) don't have a good track record for effectiveness, and they may cause visual discomfort at least or be less safe for the eyes (per a report by France's food, environmental and occupational safety agency) at worst.

- *Full-spectrum light, which mimics the color of sunlight, is not necessary.* If you like the color better, go for it, but it is no more effective and no healthier (despite claims to the contrary) than ordinary fluorescent light.

- *Higher lux (intensity up to 10,000 lux) is better.* Fixtures providing 2,500 lux have been found effective in research, but those providing closer to 10,000 give the same benefits with shorter daily exposure.

- *Size matters.* Most studies have used boxes with a one-foot-square light-emitting area. Smaller boxes are usually cheaper and take up less space, but they naturally emit less light and have to be angled correctly to ensure that the light enters your eyes. (At least one company, however, offers pairs of smaller boxes so that you can place one on either side of the surface you're sitting at so that you get your therapy "in stereo," as it were.)

- *UV light can harm the eyes and the skin.* Make sure your light box notes that most UV rays are blocked out (usually with a filter in the plastic diffuser).

⚠ Don't Try This at Home . . .

The components of a light box seem pretty simple, so people have asked me if they could just put one together on their own to save money and make it the size that will work best for them. I always say that theoretically they could, but unless they include everything a commercial fixture has, it could end up ineffective or, worse, dangerous. Omitting the plastic diffuser screen and UV filter as one person did, for example, could result in damaging your eyes.

Light fixtures seem to be coming down in price (but never buy for low price if a manufacturer lacks a track record and the unit doesn't have the features listed on page 117). You also may be able to get your insurance company to pay for at least part of the cost if you send your receipt and a letter from your doctor stating the medical necessity for light therapy to the company's claim department. A sample of a letter your doctor might send is on the facing page.

Sample Letter for Insurance Reimbursement

To Whom It May Concern:

This is to certify that Ms. Jane Smith has been a patient of mine since _____. I have treated her for recurrent major depressions (DSM-5 296.30), with a seasonal pattern. This condition, also known as seasonal affective disorder (SAD), has been shown in many studies in the United States and elsewhere in the world to respond to treatment with bright environmental light (light therapy). Light therapy is no longer considered experimental but is a mainstream type of psychiatric treatment, as evidenced by its inclusion in the authoritative *Treatments of Psychiatric Disorders, Third Edition,* a publication of American Psychiatric Publishing.[a] The effectiveness of light therapy was further confirmed in a 2005 meta-analysis published in the prestigious *American Journal of Psychiatry.*[b] To administer light therapy adequately, a light box, such as the one named in the attached invoice, is required.

Although a light box is an expensive piece of equipment, the experience of clinicians who have used it for many patients indicates that it saves a great deal of money over time by reducing the number of doctors' visits and the costs of medications and laboratory investigations of persistent symptoms, as well as the indirect costs of lost productivity. I maintain that in Ms. Smith's case, the use of such a light fixture should be regarded not only as a medical necessity, to be used in preference to, or in addition to, other forms of treatment, but also as a means of reducing her overall medical costs.

---

[a]Oren, D. A., and Rosenthal, N. E. (2001). Light therapy. In G. O. Gabbard (Ed.), *Treatments of psychiatric disorders* (3rd ed., Vol. 2, pp. 1295–1306). Washington, DC: American Psychiatric Publishing.

[b]Golden, R. N., Gaynes, B. N., Ekstrom, R. D., Hamer, R. M., Jacobsen, F. M., Suppes, T., et al. (2005). The efficacy of light therapy in the treatment of mood disorders: A review and meta-analysis of the evidence. *American Journal of Psychiatry, 162*(4), 656–662.

Reprinted with permission from *Winter Blues: Everything You Need to Know to Beat Seasonal Affective Disorder* (4th ed.), by Norman E. Rosenthal. Copyright 2013 by Norman E. Rosenthal.

If you don't think you need professional help—use the list on page 36 in Chapter 2 to make that decision, but always be open to seeking help if you have any doubts— you can try light therapy on your own and see how it works for you. Limit this trial to 2 weeks and don't hesitate to contact a doctor or therapist if you have troubling side effects, questions, or get no (or little) benefit and need further help for your SAD symptoms.

You're ready to start light therapy once you've checked off all the items on this list:

☐ I have a light box that has all the features listed in the box on page 117.

☐ I've found a place to set up the box where I'll enjoy using it every day.

☐ I have room there to set it up so that the appropriate amount of light hits my eyes.

☐ I've figured out a time in early morning when I can use it without sacrificing another important part of my daily routine.

☐ I've given some thought to what I might do while receiving light therapy that will allow me to face the light with eyes open (ideas are listed on page 122).

As soon as you receive your light fixture, enter the last date on which you can return the unit and get your money back so you don't forget:

My money-back guarantee ends on _____.

True or False? You can get light therapy while you sleep by timing your light fixture to go on before you wake up in the morning.

False. For light therapy to be effective you must:

☑ Face the box.

☑ Be within the range specified by the manufacturer.

☑ **Have your eyes open.**

While there is some interesting evidence that light may also be somewhat effective when it enters the ear, it's the eyes that have it (*it* being the research and track record) where SAD solutions are concerned. Another tool that might help if you

Treat

Creating Your Own Summer Sunrise

Why wait for summer to light up your day at 5:00 or 6:00 in the morning? Especially if you can't stand to get up that early to start light therapy, you may benefit from a dawn-simulating device, which will mimic sunup by gradually lighting up your bedroom over 30 to 60 minutes, just like a natural dawn but using artificial light, at a preset time. Although new products are always coming on the market, there are basically two types of models:

- The model that can be plugged into any incandescent lamp, allowing you to set the time for "dawn" to start and how long you want the gradual sunrise to take. This is a great aid for travelers, small enough to fit into your palm. Make sure to use a 60- to 100-watt bulb in your lamp; brighter might wake you up too suddenly.

- The self-contained model, which typically combines an alarm clock and light and doesn't need to be plugged into a lamp. You may have trouble positioning the light ideally to shine on your face when you already have a bedside lamp, but there is currently at least one small, traveling model that might work for you in that case. Many people like this all-in-one solution.

want to get therapy while sleeping is a dawn simulator—see the box above—and the dawn simulator *does* work while you're asleep and your eyes are closed.

True or False? You can sit as far away from the light box as you want, as long as the light is aimed at your eyes.

False. The farther away you are, the less the antidepressant effect. Follow your light box's directions; usually you want to be 1 to 3 feet from the light source.

Fitting Light Therapy Seamlessly into Your Life

When finding a slot for light therapy, the most critical factor is when the light therapy will be most effective, which for most people is the early morning. How can you schedule your therapy during that time period in a way that won't make it just another chore?

If getting light therapy while you take care of some obligation will motivate you—that is, if you're a person who feels good about multitasking—try these ideas:

- Save paperwork—bill paying, checkbook balancing, correspondence, list making—for first thing every morning and turn on your light box while doing it.

- Make business and consumer calls while sitting in front of the light.

- Catch up on e-mails.

- Do Internet searches (for your next winter vacation spot!).

- Fold laundry or do your ironing or mending. (May work best with a freestanding fixture where you can adjust the height of the fixture and vary the distance between you and the light source.)

- Chop food for upcoming meals.

- Buy several light boxes (if affordable) and install them in different places in your home so you can move from chore to chore (interrupting your exposure to the light for a minute while you change locations won't diminish the therapeutic effect).

If light therapy is likely to feel like another burden, try combining it with an enjoyable activity:

- Read a novel or a magazine.

- Listen to your favorite music or watch a movie on TV or your computer.

- Give yourself a manicure.

- Catch up on phone calls with friends and family you like talking to.

- Enjoy a leisurely breakfast.

- *Try setting up your light box in front of an exercise machine (works best with a freestanding unit) to get double the benefit (light + exercise; see Chapter 10)!*

Remember, what makes light therapy fit into your life seamlessly will vary from day to day depending on how you feel. On some mornings getting something done during therapy might be the best way to head off stress. On others a pleasant activity might be a better choice.

Treat

GETTING STARTED

Step 1

Set up your light fixture where you plan to use it the night before starting light therapy.

☐ **Done**

Step 2

Set your alarm if you need to. It's best to get light therapy as early as possible, so if getting up at 7:00 won't give you enough time to incorporate therapy into your schedule, consider getting up earlier—a much better choice than postponing therapy until later in the day. If you're having difficulty waking up, a dawn simulator can be a huge help; see page 121 for more on this.

Time I will start light therapy each morning: _____

I'll need to set my alarm: Yes _____ **No** _____

I'll use a dawn simulator: Yes _____ **No** _____

Step 3

If your SAD symptoms are just beginning, start with 20 minutes of therapy a day for a week and then evaluate, but always pay attention to your reactions to the therapy to figure out how much you need. You can use the typical signs that light therapy is working (listed on page 128) and the signs that you're getting too much light (page 128) as benchmarks for adjusting the amount of light you get, but everyone is unique, and sharp awareness of your own responses is key. Examples of how a few people with SAD have gauged the best duration of therapy for themselves are in the box on page 125. If you're not experiencing any bothersome side effects, keep it up for another week. If your symptoms are easing, keep up this therapeutic schedule. If you're starting later in the season and your symptoms are peaking, try 20 minutes twice a day for just a few days and then evaluate. If you're not having any side effects, add 10 minutes a day to each session until you're at 45 minutes twice a day. To get a clear picture of how well the therapy is working for you, try to stay at this schedule for a full 2 weeks and then evaluate. Use the evaluation form on page 129 to assess the benefits.

> **I'm starting therapy on _____. (This could be the date when it's convenient based on your having picked up this book or the date that you filled in, if you're planning ahead, on page 81 of Chapter 5.)**
>
> **I'm starting with 20 minutes _____ once a day (check) or _____ twice a day (check).**
>
> **I will evaluate on _____ (date).**

Step 4

If you do notice any discomfort before the trial time period is over, follow the troubleshooting directions on page 131 that apply to the problems you're experiencing.

> **I need to check out these problems:**
>
> _____
>
> _____

Step 5

As your low season rolls on, be prepared to adjust your light therapy. If you have already had a chance to plot Your SAD Graph (see Chapter 5), you can use that to give you an idea of when you might need to increase or decrease light therapy time periods based on your personal seasonality curve.

> **Based on what I know about when my symptoms increase or decrease, I'll be sure to assess whether I should start adding to therapy or cutting back on _____ (date).**

Be Aware

IS IT WORKING?

There may be nothing more important to eliminating SAD from your life than becoming intimately familiar with your day-by-day—even hour-by-hour—reaction to the seasons and to the interventions, preventive efforts, and remedies you incorporate into your treatment. Toward that end, I encourage

How Much Light Therapy to Get: Be Your Own Gauge

Only you can tell how light therapy is affecting you, so let your own experience be your guide, as these people did:

Sylvia started out with 20 minutes of light therapy at around 9:00 A.M., after getting her daughter off to school. After a week she was ready to return her light box for a refund, because her symptoms seemed exactly the same as before initiating therapy. The next day her daughter was home from school and Sylvia sat in front of the light box while drinking her coffee at 7:00 A.M. The difference was significant—she felt energized (more than she ordinarily would from coffee alone), eager about getting started on her day, and found herself humming while she tidied her apartment. She quickly realized that getting her therapy earlier boosted its benefits. But on most mornings she was too busy with her 5-year-old to fit in 20 minutes of therapy early in the day. Although she might have gotten the maximum benefit from fitting in therapy at 7:00 every morning, no one was available to help out with Janey then. She decided to try 30 minutes at 9:00. The additional time seemed to help—not as much as the earlier time slot, but enough that she was satisfied, especially since she found she could fit in another 30 minutes in the evening, while her daughter was playing.

Tom generally took a "more is better" attitude toward life, and so he started out with 30 minutes of light therapy right after getting out of bed (generally at 6:00 A.M.). At first he was excited by how much better he felt. He even found himself getting things done—paying bills, reading over a report from work—during the early morning hours when he usually felt groggy and slow. But after a few days he recognized that this new energy and focus came at a price: irritable and antsy, he found himself honking at and swerving around drivers who were "in the way" on his ride to the office and sometimes arrived with a headache. This went on for a week before Tom connected his aggravated mood with light therapy and decided to cut down to 10 minutes. Trial and error revealed that 10 minutes was too little (he went back to being sluggish in the morning) and that 15 or 20 minutes was just about right.

(cont.)

How Much Light Therapy to Get: Be Your Own Gauge (*cont.*)

Julio started light therapy in December, close to the winter solstice, and quickly discovered that he needed a full 45 minutes in front of his lights twice a day. Thrilled with being able to "avoid total hibernation" around the holidays for the first time in several years, he committed to making these light sessions a top priority. So much so that when March started to "go out like a lamb," Julio chalked up the restlessness he felt on some days, and a dryness in his eyes, to spending too much time at his computer. He kept up his 45-minute light sessions until his wife asked him why he was so tightly wound. When he thought about how much longer and brighter the days were now than they had been at the beginning of his light therapy, Julio decided his SAD season must be over and he should quit light therapy. Within 2 days he was dragging himself out of bed and getting to work late, where he couldn't focus fully on the day's tasks until he'd downed three cups of coffee. Julio realized the only way to figure out what was the appropriate amount of light therapy was to pay attention to how he felt throughout the day as sunset got later and later and also to how a particular amount of light therapy made him feel immediately afterward.

Monica has summer SAD. For years, watching those around her bask happily in the balmy weather while she felt agitated and moody only compounded her blues. Desperate for an antidote, she speculated that her summer depression might be related to unstable circadian rhythms, a condition that often responds to pulses of early-morning light. Monica started getting up at dawn and going outside in the sun for a few minutes. Within a few days of this routine she was much more inclined to frolic with everyone else who was enjoying the long, warm days. Still, she knew this remedy was her own personal experiment, and there was no predicting how it would work going forward. The only thing she could do was monitor her own reactions closely: If she stopped getting into the sunlight at 5:30, she discovered her symptoms came roaring back within a couple days. And as summer shifted to fall, she found she could start phasing out her early-morning sunlight treatments.

you to use the Daily Mood Log in Chapter 6 to record how you feel every day and what measures you took to ease SAD symptoms. There's no better way to get the complete picture of what's helping, alone or in combination with something else.

If you're just starting to use your SAD Solution APP, however, and light therapy is the first tool you're trying, you might find it simpler to start by just filling out the Monitoring Light Therapy form on page 129 for your trial period. The information you record can help you consider whether you need to change the amount of light therapy, add another type of treatment, or address side effects. Forms like this one give you a simple mechanism for tuning in to your own mind and body and using what you learn to get the most out of a remedy. You don't have to give a lot of thought to your reactions to the light therapy. Just jot down how you feel afterward and then review what you've recorded later. Feeling a little sluggish over the last few days? Take a look at your log and see whether you notice a link between changes in energy and changes in your light therapy routine. If so, you know it's time to try more light therapy. Feeling too revved up? Maybe you're getting too much light and should cut back a bit.

If you find this kind of information gathering helpful, feel free to make extra copies of the form to use it beyond the trial period and learn how light affects you as the weeks and months progress. Many people with SAD don't immediately realize when symptoms are creeping back. This log gives you a way to step outside of yourself and see possible connections that may be clouded by SAD symptoms. It's easy to attribute feeling lousy to external events. Having a way to look objectively at your light therapy experience may help you see that SAD and light are at the root of low mood, not what's happening in your life and world. That's good news, because how much light therapy you get is under your control!

Be Aware • Use Monitoring Forms Like Training Wheels

The beauty of monitoring forms and planning tools is not that they are useful records. It's that you won't need them forever. As your brain draws the connections between a remedy you try and how you feel afterward, you hone the instinct to manage your own SAD without the record keeping. Use the monitoring forms whenever they feel helpful, and eventually you'll find yourself adjusting your SAD solution APP without even putting the need for a change into words, much less on paper.

★ KEY POINTS

Signs to Watch For

Over time you'll become acutely aware of how light therapy is affecting you—when you get too little, you'll notice your symptoms starting to creep back; too much, and you'll feel like you've had too much coffee, or you may suffer some of the other side effects listed below that you don't experience when the effects you notice are all good. Here are the kinds of things you may notice when you start to use light therapy. You can check off the ones you experience here or use the list for reference and enter them when you notice them in the monitoring form on the facing page.

- ☐ Lightness in your body
- ☐ Tranquility
- ☐ Increased energy
- ☐ Butterflies in your stomach
- ☐ Pins and needles in your hands
- ☐ Chores don't feel like *huge* chores
- ☐ Decreased sleepiness
- ☐ Fewer carb cravings
- ☐ Clear mind
- ☐ Brighter mood
- ☐ Increased sociability
- ☐ Increased sex drive

⚠ *Ouch!*

Intolerable side effects from light therapy are very rare, but mild versions of the ones listed below call for some kind of change to ameliorate discomfort so you can still reap the benefits.

- ☐ **Headaches**
- ☐ **Eye strain**
- ☐ **Irritability/anxiety**
- ☐ **Overactivity**
- ☐ **Insomnia**
- ☐ **Nausea**
- ☐ **Fatigue**
- ☐ **Dry eyes**

Monitoring Light Therapy

Be Aware

Fill out this form as often as you can after using light therapy. This form has space for 21 days of recording. Make copies or download the form from *www.guilford. com/rosenthal3-forms* to print out extras if you want to extend your monitoring. Be sure to enter information for both therapy sessions if you're getting light therapy twice a day. Use the Notes column to record thoughts about any changes your experience that day might warrant or how you felt the time and setting worked for you.

Light fixture(s) used: _____

_____

Light intensity: _____ lux

Distance from light source: _____ feet

Date	Time(s)	Positive Effects	Side Effects	Notes

(cont.)

Monitoring Light Therapy (cont.)

Date	Time(s)	Positive Effects	Side Effects	Notes

☐ **Dry nasal passages/sinuses**

☐ **Sunburn-type skin reaction**

┃▲┃ SCIENCE

Light therapy has been shown in research <u>NOT</u> to be harmful to:

- pregnant women

- pets

- children*

- the eyes*

- the skin*

TROUBLESHOOTING: WHAT TO DO WHEN PROBLEMS ARISE

If you're not getting any positive effects after a week of light therapy (or a few days if it's the middle of your blue season), check out the following:

- Are you getting light early enough in the day? One study found that light therapy was twice as effective (response rate going from 40–80%) when people shifted to an earlier time.

    Possible solution: Try shifting your therapy half an hour to an hour earlier for a few days and see if that helps. If not, keep going earlier until you get a benefit or you can't stand to get up that early.

- Is the box in the appropriate therapeutic position—at the distance recommended by the manufacturer and oriented at eye level?

---

*Infants' eyes are much more sensitive to light than adults', so make sure your baby—and ideally any child under age 10—is not staring directly at the lights while you use them. There is no evidence of danger to the eyes from using a good-quality light box, nor is there evidence of skin damage. But if you have had an unusual eye disease or condition, see your eye doctor before starting light therapy. Similarly, light therapy is unlikely to cause any skin problems, but if you have had skin cancer, consult your doctor before starting therapy. For those with fair or sensitive skin, I recommend sunblock on the face to protect it from the small amount of UV light that might elude the filters built into light fixtures. (Remember, the best sunblock works against both UVA and UVB.)

Possible solution: If you can't move it closer in its current location, check the list of possible other activities during which you can get light therapy and see whether one of those locations will work better.

- Is enough light coming from the box?

   Possible solution: If you're trying one of the smaller boxes (less than a foot square), you might not be able to get enough light. Try extending the duration of your exposure or adding an evening session. Or get a bigger light.

- Are you giving it too little time?

   Possible solution: Increase your session to 45 minutes or use a 30-minute morning session and 15 minutes in the evening.

If you're still not getting any benefit (or enough benefit) after 2 weeks at 45 minutes twice a day, you may need to replace or augment light therapy. See the rest of Part II of this book and also consult your doctor.

If you're noticing side effects while you also get positive effects, check out the following:

- Are you feeling antsy or amped up?

   Possible solution: You may be getting too much light. Some people can get a benefit from only 5 to 10 minutes a day, and anything more will make them uncomfortable. This may be particularly true for those who have a history of mania or hypomania. Try cutting back to 10 to 15 minutes of light therapy a day and then gradually building back up over the next week or two or moving a little farther away from the light source until you feel better and then try moving back closer to get the full benefit of light.

⚠ **Use light therapy only under the supervision of a doctor if you have a history of bipolar disorder.**

Those with a history of bipolar disorder must take special care with light therapy since it can trigger mania:

- **Involve your doctor from the beginning.**

- **Use no more than 5 minutes of light therapy to start with.**

- **With no side effects after a week or so, try another 5 minutes.**

- Are you feeling anxious, irritable, or restless?

     Possible solution: If cutting back on light doesn't alleviate the symptoms, consult your doctor immediately.

- Are you having trouble sleeping after using light therapy?

     Possible solution: This usually happens after evening light therapy, so try moving your session earlier in the day or even earlier in the evening.

- Are you feeling nauseated?

     Possible solution: Sometimes this comes with anxiety caused by light therapy, but according to one researcher, it's those who are getting positive effects who usually have this side effect, so I encourage you to try cutting back just a little on the therapy so you don't miss out on its benefits.

- Are you feeling tired?

     Possible solution: If this is the result of getting up earlier to get light therapy, as it frequently is, try going to bed earlier. If that doesn't work, you might have to move your therapy to later in the morning, which is less than ideal.

- Do your eyes or nose feel dry?

     Possible solution: Light boxes put out dry heat, so consider using a humidifier while getting light therapy or drinking something hot, like tea. If you wear contacts, dryness can cause corneal abrasions, so try using artificial tears—or put in your contacts after your light therapy.

- Do you feel like you're getting a sunburn?

     Possible solution: Use sunblock, especially if you have pale or sensitive skin.

If you've started to get less benefit after lots of improvement, check out the following:

- Has your stress increased?

     Possible solution: Use the strategies in Chapter 9 to examine your stress level and address any new stresses added to your life.

- Is it gloomier outside or are you going deeper into the winter?

    Possible solution: Try increasing your light therapy. Sometimes midwinter is cloudier than late fall and the ambient light has diminished, calling for a countermeasure of more therapy.

- Have a couple years passed since you started light therapy?

    Possible solution: Sometimes fluorescent bulbs lose their intensity over time, although you often won't be able to detect this because it happens gradually. If your bulbs haven't been replaced in two winters, consider buying new ones.

WHAT HAVE YOU LEARNED FROM LIGHT THERAPY?

Sometimes writing down what you gained (or where your expectations weren't met) helps gel your thoughts and stimulate new ideas. If you think it might help you plan for next year, jot down some notes at the end of winter about what you got out of light therapy, anything you want to change, and any side effects to address.

_____

_____

_____

_____

_____

_____

_____

    Adding this information to your action plan in Chapter 6 can keep it useful as an up-to-date reference.

8

More Light

Brightening Your Environment, at Home and Away

★ KEY POINTS

Did light therapy work well for you?

If so, then you might get even more help if you try the easy self-help methods in this chapter to give you a boost all year.

If not, you might want to move on to try the tools in the following chapters—but see the information on negative ions in this chapter too.

Be Aware

WHAT DO YOU HOPE TO GET OUT OF ADDING LIGHT TO YOUR ENVIRONMENT?

☐ I hope more light will take care of the symptoms that light therapy didn't alleviate.

☐ I hope extra environmental light will enable me to get by with shorter light therapy sessions.

☐ I hope boosting environmental light early in the year will postpone the onset of my symptoms each year.

☐ I hope to discover whether a vacation from the dark and cold will be worth the expense.

In Chapter 4 you rated your interest in adding light to your home and/or workspace and taking a winter vacation to a sunnier location. Now that you've undergone a trial of light therapy, how would you rate your interest?

Adding light to my home _____

Adding light to my workspace _____

Taking a winter vacation _____

If your ratings are the same as or higher than they were when you worked through Chapter 4, get started! It's best to plan and make these changes while your energy is high, probably in spring or summer, to benefit from them when you need them most, probably in fall and winter.

⚠ ***Those with summer SAD (without winter SAD) don't need to add light to their environment.***

In fact, some people have found lowering their indoor light helpful, although there is no research evidence to back this up. We don't know whether summer SAD is related to changes in light or temperature. Staying in a cool indoor space a lot of the time has helped some people, but again, we have no scientific studies to show how commonly useful this remedy is.

ADDING LIGHT TO YOUR HOME

↗ **FAST FACTS**

- More light is better: any way you add light to your environment helps replace waning daylight.

- Permanent changes that will let in a lot more light include enlarging windows, adding new ones, or installing skylights or other light from above.

- Temporary changes (ideal when you're renting your home or living in someone else's home) include choosing decor like bright, light-colored pictures or curtains.

- What's outside matters: Trimming foliage around windows and making sure only deciduous trees and shrubs are near windows ensures that light won't be blocked in the crucial winter months.

- Cleaning grime off windows can make a surprising difference to a room.
- Full-spectrum lights in your house may be more pleasing but are probably no more therapeutic than regular incandescent or fluorescent light bulbs.

Treat

Doing a Home Light Inspection

Are you getting as much light in your home as you could? A good way to find out is by doing a thorough light inspection. It may feel easiest to do this inspection during the season when you have the most energy, but in some cases the information you need can be gained only during your low season, so you might want to do this inspection in summer and then review in winter.

Step 1

List the rooms in your home to the left of the colon in the blanks below. Place an asterisk next to the rooms you spend the most time in, with a D if you spend most of your time there during the day and an N if at night or in the evening (while awake).

_____ : _____

_____

_____

_____ . _____

_____

_____

_____ : _____

_____

_____

_____ : _____

_____

_____ : _____

_____

_____

_____: _____

_____

_____

Step 2

Now take a thorough tour of each room, noting after the colon in each blank above where and how much light is available, both natural and artificial. Picture yourself in the places where you usually sit, stand, or engage in some activity and evaluate the light that strikes your face there. (This is a case where the angle of the light matters most in winter.)

Step 3

Decide what kinds of changes you could make to increase light in each spot, paying particular attention to the rooms you spend the most time in and noting whether you could add natural light (if you spend daytime hours there) or artificial (if you spend evening hours there or you could augment natural light during the day with artificial). Get creative and specific (for example, "Move the floor lamp that's near the wall right next to the chair where I usually read") and list as many ideas as you can in the blanks above. Refer to "22 Ways to Brighten Your Home" on the facing page if you're feeling uninspired. Don't worry about how practical the ideas are right now; you don't have to commit to any of them right away.

Step 4

Start with making the changes that seem likely to reap the greatest benefits at the least cost and cross them off as you make them.

Step 5

Try to repeat your inspection tour during the opposite season of the year (if you're doing it in spring or summer, repeat in winter and vice versa) to take into account seasonal needs as the length of the day changes.

⚠️ *If you're about to buy or rent a new home . . .*

Try to find out how the changes of season will affect the light entering your new home. As mentioned in Chapter 4, evergreens that provide a welcome privacy screen in the

summer may block out the sun in winter. A bedroom that faces west may keep the summer sunrise from pushing you out of bed before you need to get up, but it may keep you in bed way past your desired waking time in the winter. A basement or first-floor apartment may seem fine in spring, but once winter comes, you might wish you had a top-floor unit with skylights instead.

Treat

⚡ 22 Ways to Brighten Your Home

1. Add tabletop and floor lamps.

2. Add ceiling fixtures or wall sconces.

3. Up the wattage in light bulbs.

4. Move lamps to shine on your face where you usually spend your time in that room.

5. Add light boxes to every room.

6. Cut skylights in ceilings (try one over your bathtub!).

7. Install SunPipes (less intrusive than skylights while providing plenty of light).

8. Move furniture so that you're facing bright windows when sitting in the room.

9. Remove curtains from windows to let in maximum light.

10. Replace opaque shades and blinds with translucent shades or gauzy fabric blinds to provide privacy without loss of much light.

11. Instead of heavy window treatments, line windowpanes with decorative translucent film—another great way to let in light but maintain privacy.

12. Paint walls white, yellow, or ivory rather than dark colors. Avoid dark paneling or wallpaper.

13. Hang paintings that contain big splashes of yellow or orange (sun colors!).

14. Make creative use of picture lights to focus spots of light on those bright paintings or even to brighten up a darker painting that you love or shine light on a bright plant or other decorative object.

15. Replace a large *dark* piece of furniture with something light or bright—a white leather sofa instead of brown, yellow or beige upholstery instead of dark patterns, light-colored woods or stains (light beech or oak versus dark mahogany).

16. **If replacement or reupholstering isn't affordable, add light, bright throws and pillows or use bright slipcovers.**

17. **Replace heavy woods, dark metals, and dark fabrics with bright metals (chrome, aluminum, gold picture frames, even polished brass) and glass.**

18. **Hang mirrors, which reflect light and can be positioned to repeat a bright feature in the room like a yellow or orange painting.**

19. **Wash windows regularly; grimy windows obscure a lot of incoming light.**

20. **Add shiny surfaces to the decor and keep them polished.**

21. **Paint and/or carpet your darkest rooms in white or other light colors.**

22. **Light candles at night to add soft light and don't hesitate to treat yourself to evenings curled up before the fire if you have a fireplace!**

> *In the ancient Chinese system of feng shui, bright yellow and orange are considered the gentler shades of the fire element represented by red, which heightens passion and energy—a good counter for depression!—while light yellows and beiges support overall health.*

⚠️ ***Don't start a remodeling project in fall!***

You probably won't have the energy to consider a major task like this during the darkest days, but some people with SAD still feel pretty good in fall and start projects that will be stressful to continue in winter or will make them feel guilty for abandoning. See Chapter 9 for more tips on managing your to-do lists and obligations to keep stress low and to avoid feeling bad for having limitations that you can't help. Chapter 14 can help you replace negative thoughts such as that you are to blame for having SAD.

If you find in November that a room you spend a lot of time in really needs more light, enlist the help of friends or family as needed to take the simplest routes—higher-wattage light bulbs, a few extra lamps, purchase of a couple of bright accents—and leave the bigger projects like repainting or refurnishing or house refitting for spring.

BRIGHTENING YOUR WORKSPACE

Unless you own your own business or are self-employed, you probably have a lot less control over your workspace than your home. But you may have more control than you think. Perhaps you are in the position to:

- Redecorate or refurnish your workspace

- Change locations within the workplace (for example, to another office, cubicle, or desk)

- Change your work shift from evenings or nights to daytime

- Transfer to a different branch, store, or other location your employer has

- Do the same job out of a home office at least for part of the week, by telecommuting

- Switch to a more SAD-friendly job within the same organization (for example, one that will get you outdoors more)

- Find a new job/employer

- Become self-employed

If you work for someone else, outside your home, it can feel difficult to ask for changes to your immediate surroundings. You may worry that it will seem as if you're asking for privileges or perks you haven't earned (a brighter office might be a perk in everyone's book!) or that you'll be embarrassed to admit that you need these accommodations to do your job well. Fortunately, many people with SAD have found that their employers are much more understanding than they might have expected.

If you're seeking only minor accommodations, such as permission to bring a light box into the workplace, you might be able to explain simply that you have "a slight case of the winter blues." Small light boxes and those designed to look like desk lamps might be sufficient. If you need a bigger light box, you'll need to take care that the light doesn't blast the person in the next cubicle. Sometimes this can be finessed easily by shifting to a cubicle that faces a wall instead of outward into the wider work area. Keep in mind that trying to work things out amicably with your supervisor and coworkers is a great stress buster.

You may very well qualify for more significant accommodations on the basis of the Americans with Disabilities Act (for more information, check the website of the U.S. Equal Employment Opportunity Commission, *www.eeoc.gov*). I have seen patients receive accommodations such as a window office or the right to telecommute.

You might not have to invoke the law, but remember that SAD is a legitimate illness that increases your need for exposure to light and you have a right to an environment that makes it possible for you to do a job for which you are otherwise qualified. Still, it's important to use your best judgment; you might want to decide whether you'll feel better overall if you try to make adjustments to your current space on your own or you approach your employer for help. Here are some options either way:

Treat

☀️ **Tips for Coping with a Dim Workspace**

- **Keep the blinds raised on any window near you if it's agreeable to coworkers exposed to the same window.**

- **Keep one (or a pair) of the smaller light boxes on your desk. Some light fixtures are designed to look like desk lamps and can therefore be used without tipping your hand about your SAD symptoms.**

- **Add a small flexible desktop lamp (like a Tensor lamp) so you can direct extra light where it will brighten your space most.**

- **Add a bright (as at home, yellows and oranges are best) poster or painting to your space.**

- **Take your coffee breaks outdoors, in the sun.**

- **Find a coworker who will go for a walk with you at lunchtime on sunny days.**

- **Scope out brightly lit restaurants or ones with lots of window-side tables if you go out to lunch.**

- **Be diligent about sticking to your morning light therapy schedule on workdays.**

How to Talk to Your Employer about Workplace Accommodations

- Stress that it's light that you need, not that prized "corner office," for the sake of your ability to do your job and for your health.

- Offer to provide a letter from your doctor stating the medical basis of your needs.

- Offer to loan your supervisor a copy of *Winter Blues* or just copy this paragraph adapted from the book if he or she is not familiar with SAD:

It can be helpful to think of SAD as similar, in certain critical ways, to a physical illness. We do not know what the underlying abnormality is in SAD, but it presumably resides somewhere in the brain, where some chemical processes do not function normally, resulting in all the symptoms of the condition. Somehow, light entering the eyes plays an important role in these key chemical processes. During the short, dark days of winter, when there is not enough light in the environment, the brain-chemical abnormality becomes manifest in the form of SAD symptoms—those relevant to work including reduced energy, difficulty concentrating and processing information, and depression. Bright light reverses the symptoms, presumably by correcting the underlying abnormality. As a diabetic needs insulin shots, your employee with SAD needs extra light and may benefit tremendously from accommodations or adaptations of the physical workplace to expose the employee to as much light as possible.

• Before asking for a different workspace, scope out possible spaces. If changing offices or cubicles would mean imposing the darker space on a coworker (which obviously most people would not like), can you suggest anything in trade? Is there a brighter space that is smaller so that the person you switch with would get the trade-off of extra room? Could you occupy a space that isn't used as office space right now, so taking it over wouldn't inconvenience a coworker?

• Think about whether it would make sense to ask a coworker with a brighter space privately whether he or she would mind switching if the boss goes along with it. Or should you leave it to your boss to negotiate? A lot depends on the nature of your workplace relationships. Do whatever feels least stressful for you.

• If you're starting to occupy a new workspace during your best time of year, that's the time to bring up the issue of light, assuming you can tell then what the space will be like at the darkest time of year. When you feel your best, you might not want to rock the boat, but that's also when you're likely to have the confidence and calm to state your case plainly, without self-doubt.

Treat

TAKING A WINTER BREAK TO SEEK THE SUN

↗ FAST FACTS

• At least a week is usually needed for a vacation to have benefits.
• Be prepared to resume treatment immediately after a vacation; the memory of light fades rapidly, and the biochemical benefits seem to stay behind when you head back north.

From November through April, resorts in the Caribbean, Central America, Mexico, and other areas that are warm and sunny are packed with visitors from the northern United States, Canada, the United Kingdom, and northern Europe. Winter can feel endless even to

> *A walk in the morning sun on a cold winter day when the ground is covered in snow can be a mini-vacation every day—another kind of light therapy.*

those who don't suffer from SAD. Why should you feel any different? Of course, winter vacations aren't always practical or affordable, but here are some ideas for arranging to head for the sun in the darkest months.

☐ Can you save up vacation time through the year to ensure that you have time for a winter break?

☐ Can you spend some time during your high-energy months checking for the best deals? The lowest rates are usually had when trips are booked far in advance, and many people with SAD report getting some relief from the creeping dread that accompanies fall when they know they have a break all set up.

☐ Consider something more exotic than the typical subtropical resort? Antarctica in the northern hemisphere's winters has almost constant sunlight.

☐ Make sure everything you need for light therapy is ready for your return. It's easy to forget you still have SAD when the biological effects of the light from a trip to a sunny place are still with you. But two or three days after returning north symptoms can return with a vengeance, so be sure to start using light as soon as you get back.

☐ Be sure you know the signs of *over*exposure to light—racing thoughts, sleeplessness, mania—in case you get too much beach or pool time, and choose a place where you can have fun even out of the sun if you need to limit your exposure periodically.

⚠ *Beware!*

On returning from a vacation in a sunny place, you may feel so good that you can forget you have SAD. That can lead to neglecting light therapy and your other anti-SAD regimen, which may result in a resounding slump. So restart your program *as soon as you get home.*

RELOCATING

Treat

⤴ FAST FACTS

- Always spend time in the winter in a new location you're considering before moving, to make sure it really does make you feel better.

- Farther south doesn't always mean brighter: How cloudy is the new location in winter? Does it have a dark monsoon season?

When gaining a lot more light is what you need and you can't seem to get it through less drastic solutions, relocating might be worth considering. But obviously such a transition demands a lot of forethought.

- Could you move to a brighter home or a brighter spot in the same community so no one in the family has to change jobs or schools as well as homes?

- Is farther south guaranteed to be better? Maybe not. If the climate is generally cloudy and rainy, it might feel just as gloomy to you as your current location farther north. Check the area's year-round climate before deciding where to look for your new home. And keep in mind that not every location within a new area will be ideal. Take Hawaii, for example: Some places are quite sunny, while others lie in the shadows of the volcanic mountains.

- If you find a sunny, warm locale, will it really be a better place to live? That depends on a lot of other factors that could affect your stress level. Is the location more remote, requiring you to do a lot more daily traveling to get where you and your family need to go? Are the social and cultural opportunities the kind that you find pleasant and stimulating? Will you know people there before you move so you'll have companionship and support? Is the cost of living there affordable? Is the terrain pleasing to you? (The desert might be sunny, but if you thrive where there's lots of water, it might not feel like the best environment.)

💡 *There may be other reasons to relocate . . .*

Even if getting more light is your top priority, managing or reducing stress can be just as important. See Chapter 9 for details and tools. On the subject of relocating, is

the place you live causing you stress outside of providing too little light? One mother I knew, Susan, found that, although she and her family adored their house in the woods, it wasn't really the shade on the property that caused a problem (they had trimmed much of the foliage to let light into the house). Rather, the fact that it was so far away from schools, stores, and places of business meant that Susan was spending half her day transporting herself and the kids from one place to the next, leaving her too little time for other obligations and virtually no time to take care of her own needs. So after seriously considering all the pros and cons, she and her husband sold their house and moved a lot closer to the center of their community. Yes, they chose a house with plenty of light. But the extra time Susan gained in her day had a significant effect on her winter symptoms—and gave her time to sit in the hot tub on their deck in the winter sun a few times a week.

It's a simple thing, but sometimes just writing down the pros and cons when you're considering a change can pave the way to the best decision. If you feel this might help you and you're thinking of relocating, a blank form to fill in with the pros and cons appears on the facing page.

NEGATIVE IONS: AS GOOD AS LIGHT THERAPY?

Treat

It sounds like science fiction, but it's not: A small machine that generates negative ions may do you as much good as light therapy. Positively charged particles like those blown around in "ill winds" such as the fabled Santa Ana winds of California have long been said to cause mental disturbances. So it made sense to speculate on whether negative ions might have the opposite effect. We already know that places full of negative ions—near water, like ocean beaches, a forest after a storm, a waterfall—make most of us feel good. So researchers Michael and Jiuan Su Terman decided to see how negative ions would affect those with SAD. They found that 30 minutes of negative ion exposure had the same antidepressant effect as 30 minutes of 10,000-lux light therapy.

What a boon to those of us who are trying to cope with SAD! If you have found light therapy effective but not a cure-all, you can augment your light therapy with use of a negative-ion generator. Or if you didn't get much from light therapy, you could try negative ions alone and see if you reap more benefits. Keep these points in mind if you decide to try a negative ion generator:

☑ **Make sure the unit you buy is a high-flow-rate generator like the one available from the Center for Environmental Therapeutics (see Resources). Gen-**

MOVE OR STAY?

Pros	Cons

erators like the air purifiers that put out a low density of negative ions are no more effective than a placebo.

☑ Do not try to use the negative ion generator and a light box at the same time or the ions may be diverted to the grounded light box.

☑ An effective generator is a fairly significant investment, so as with light boxes, make sure you know the return policy should you need to get your money back.

SCIENCE

See the Resources section at the back of the book for information on ordering a negative ion generator.

WHAT HAVE YOU LEARNED FROM ADDING MORE LIGHT?

Sometimes writing down what you gained (or where your expectations weren't met) helps gel your thoughts and stimulate new ideas. If you think it might help you plan for next year, jot down any thoughts about additional environmental changes and winter vacation plans you want to make.

_____

_____

_____

_____

_____

_____

_____

_____

Adding this information to your action plan in Chapter 6 can keep it useful as an up-to-date reference.

9

Lightening the Load

Acceptance, Stress Management, and Support

Now that you've considered and applied some strategies for adding light to your life, how do you feel?

☐ I'm proud that I've done something for myself in an attempt to feel better. It wasn't easy, but I did it.

☐ I feel grateful every day that those around me have been so understanding and supportive.

☐ I don't always like myself that much, and being reminded that others care gives me a real boost.

☐ I feel stronger. I can see how every change I've made to get more light has made me feel a little bit better, and this makes me feel like I could do even more.

☐ I have hope for my future: If I can make the inroads I've already made into my SAD symptoms, I might be able to live the kind of life I want year-round from now on.

Acceptance, Stress Management, and Support Can Help with Summer SAD Too

Although no controlled studies have been done to show that nonpharmacological treatments work for summer SAD (there is some anecdotal evidence that staying cool or out of direct sunlight helps), there's little doubt that those with the summer syndrome could benefit from the help found in this chapter.

> ### Be Aware

If you got any benefit from light, I hope you were able to check off at least a couple of the statements on page 149. But in reality, many people with SAD still have difficulty accepting that they have a biologically based chronic illness. Do you ever experience any of the following?

☐ **I feel a little embarrassed when people come into my home and ask what my light boxes are.**

☐ **I'm chagrined at having to ask for the brightest possible space at work.**

☐ **I feel guilty asking my family to take our vacations in winter when I know they've always enjoyed summer beach and camping trips.**

☐ **Sometimes having a disorder makes me feel damaged, or like a lesser human being compared to those around me—a burden to others and to myself.**

Having any chronic illness is hard on morale. But because some people with seasonal symptoms believe they *should not* be affected by these inevitable annual shifts, they may struggle with shame, guilt, and self-blame. If this is true for you, try to take this first section of the chapter to heart. Accepting that you have an illness that is not your fault can open the door to getting the maximum benefit from any tool or treatment you decide to try.

> ### Prevent

HOW ACCEPTING SAD CAN GIVE YOU POWER OVER IT

It's perfectly natural to feel sad about having SAD—even when extra light is starting to open a window of hope for you. The trouble is, feelings of regret, shame, guilt, and even anger about being oppressed by the change of seasons tend to immobilize us, rob us of mental and physical energy, and feed on themselves.

A major goal of this book is to give you small, manageable ways to make incremental improvements in your symptoms. Feeling better feeds on itself too. The weaker your symptoms become, the stronger your ability to stick to the interventions that work for you and to fine-tune your regimen to loosen SAD's grip further. So before you dig any deeper into the SAD toolkit in this book, it may be important to ask yourself how fully you've accepted having SAD and having to integrate the limitations it imposes into your life.

☐ **Do you sometimes skip your light therapy because "it's just silly" that you need it?**

☐ **Do you avoid family and friends when you're feeling your worst because you're sure they'll be disappointed in your inability to "cheer up"?**

☐ **Have you stuck with holiday traditions that you've begun to dread because it's too hard to explain that you're not up to hosting or going out?**

☐ **When you feel angry about having SAD, does your anger often end up directed at yourself?**

☐ **Do you hate having to explain what SAD is, sure you'll be met with disbelief?**

These are some of the signs of having difficulty accepting SAD and the limitations it imposes. But before you start beating yourself up for lack of acceptance, understand that acceptance comes slowly. Being faced with someone else's skepticism is never going to be enjoyable, but in time and with appropriate treatment you will come to the conviction that you have a biologically based illness, it's not your fault, you really do feel worse at certain times of year, and you may have to cut back on what you're expected to do during those times.

Until that day comes, you may find that keeping your light boxes out of the sight of strangers spares you questions you don't feel like answering right now . . . that it feels easier to keep to your tradition of hosting a New Year's Day buffet than it would be to worry about disappointing people . . . that it's okay to avoid *some* phone calls when you're really not up to talking. Sometimes you know who your true friends are by seeing who accepts your limitations and difficulties (and let's face it, we all have some). It's all about figuring out what is going to cause you the most stress while you're coming to terms with this problem you never asked for. (And, as we have already done in Part I of this book, we will continue to take the liberty of reminding you that having SAD is not your fault because we know how easy it is to lose hold of that conviction.)

Treat

And whenever your anger about having SAD shifts from being mad at the world to beating *yourself* up, try to call up this mantra:

Having SAD is not my fault.

If you think it might help, write that down on a notecard to keep in your pocket, enter it into your smartphone, add it to your screen saver, or post it on your bathroom mirror. Any time you feel beaten down by seasonal depression or embarrassed or ashamed because you can't be the same person in winter that you are at other times of year, pull out your card or your phone or shift from whatever you are doing on your computer to the desktop where that message is stored.

If you're new to the diagnosis of SAD, you might also print out the list of facts on the facing page and post them where you can see them regularly. While you're finding the best way to deal with SAD's restrictions, just do whatever feels like the best you can do and always aim for prevention. If you can't bear to let go of your tradition of having your extended family over for Christmas Eve, try to plan for help ahead of time. Maybe you make it a potluck, or assign everyone a dish to bring. Or hire someone to spend a few hours setting up the party for you. Plan to accept everyone's offer of helping you clean up afterward. You might be surprised by the fact that pitching in makes everyone feel good while it's also relieving you of extra stress. Whatever works well can be continued next year, and things that are less successful will give you ideas for planning next year's event.

 Have you had to make any tough decisions like this? If so, jot down below any ideas you have for sowing the seeds for change before winter arrives next year (or, if you feel like it, go back to Chapter 6 and jot those ideas down in the blanks supplied for the appropriate season):

_____

_____

_____

I think of acceptance as one leg of a tripod that supports resilience and therefore strengthens all your other efforts to reduce SAD's effects. The other two legs are stress management and support. On these three legs rests your ability to maximize the benefits of all kinds of beneficial treatments and self-help strategies.

How you might use the power of acceptance:

- **You'll find ways to set reasonable goals for yourself in winter so you feel good about what you get done even at the hardest time of year.**

Having SAD Is Nothing to Be Ashamed Of

Being affected by the change of seasons doesn't make me weird or different:

- About 5% of the U.S. population has SAD.

- Another 14% has milder seasonal symptoms.

I came by it honestly:

- SAD or some other form of depression runs in many families.

- My symptoms may have multiplied thanks to my living at a northern latitude.

I'm not making up how bad I feel in the winter (or summer):

- I've tried to ignore my seasonal symptoms, but that doesn't make them go away.

- There is no way I would ever want to feel this bad.

SAD is true depression:

- It's a disorder recognized by psychiatrists around the world.

- It can't be controlled by sheer willpower.

It is important to do whatever it takes to ease my symptoms:

- I wouldn't ask a diabetic to do without insulin just because I don't have diabetes.

- I wouldn't expect someone to just "get over" needing glasses to see.

- I would never ask someone with a chronic medical illness to "just live with it" instead of trying to feel better.

- Helping myself feel better may be the nicest thing I can do for those around me, because it will make me more pleasant to be around, more productive, and more able to do things for others.

- **You'll get the help you need in winter even though you know you can handle these things on your own in summer—because you have a right to get help for a problem that isn't your fault.**

- **You'll stick to your light therapy schedule because you'll know the benefits are real and the setbacks you'll suffer by skipping therapy for a few days are disproportionate to any time "saved."**

- **You'll stop denying yourself mood-boosting activities in favor of catching up on the obligations that SAD has prevented you from meeting.**

- **You'll feel freer to be with those who provide energizing companionship and support because you know they won't demand that you act like your spring and summer self.**

- **You won't postpone consulting a doctor or therapist on the theory that your symptoms are bearable and will just go away if you ignore them.**

- **You'll feel more comfortable saying no when you need to.**

- **You'll be able to explain SAD to the uninitiated without feeling sheepish or defensive.**

What you might gain as a result of these shifts: social support, reduced stress, self-esteem, energy conservation, and maximum treatment benefits.

Treat　　Like any tripod, your SAD solution tripod is likely to wobble a little if all three legs aren't pretty sturdy. Acceptance is best developed when you have the support of others, but you're also likely to get acceptance, followed by support, from others once *you've* accepted SAD. Stress lowers your resilience and can leave you vulnerable to self-blame, which can discourage you from seeking support from others. Their interdependence is the reason these three issues are discussed together in this chapter. But you'll discover that the interdependence of effective treatments goes even further. Here, for example, are some ideas for how you can boost acceptance with the help of tools in later chapters:

Lack of acceptance is often based in negative thoughts and questionable beliefs.

- Turn to Chapter 14 to learn how to systematically challenge and replace automatic thoughts that keep you stuck in shame, blame, and denial—the habits of thinking that build a wall between you and your SAD Solution APP.

Science has shown that self-esteem, which can fuel the pursuit of health and happiness, is based largely on competence. Initiative is awfully hard to take when you're depressed, and it becomes even harder if you set unrealistic goals and then feel you've failed when they elude you. But if you take small steps to build new skills to ease your symptoms, you'll gain self-confidence and self-esteem.

- Turn to Chapter 11 to take control of your diet if you're down on yourself for gaining weight every winter and to boost physical activity. Exercise offers a multitude of benefits that are hard to believe until you experience them, which you will almost the minute you start exercising (and exercise is a way to "get out there" without having to talk to anyone if you find it tough to get going in the morning, like many people with SAD).

- Turn to Chapter 12 to learn meditation, a powerful way to gain self-acceptance and a scientifically proven benefit to those with SAD.

- Try reinforcing your accomplishments by doing the little exercise below. Giving yourself credit for the little things you do sharpens your awareness of your efforts and your achievements and can encourage you to keep up the good work.

Be Aware

Don't let pride or prejudice stand in your way of considering medication. People's attitudes toward medication can be complicated. Some people resist medication because they associate it with a label of "mental illness," which they find uncomfortable. Others tell themselves if they can't solve their problem by other routes, they are "weak." Still others fear that once they start taking medication they'll be dependent on it for life. These misperceptions are tangled up in lack of acceptance as both cause and effect. If you try the self-help methods in this book and still suffer disabling symptoms, don't hesitate to talk to a prescriber.

- Turn to Chapter 14 and try to challenge your beliefs about medication if you've tried everything else and still hesitate to seek medicine for depression.

- Turn to Chapter 15 for facts and figures about medication for SAD. If medication ends up working for you, what more proof do you need that you have a biological illness that isn't your fault?

Giving Yourself Credit

When depressed, it's easy to focus on the negatives in your day, such as what you haven't gotten done. It's also common to drift through mundane tasks in a fog and not really remember what you've managed to do. Therefore some people find it helpful to remind themselves that they've accomplished more during a day than they ordinarily give themselves credit for. Try to allow yourself to register your accomplishments, no matter how small they may seem at the time. You can give yourself a little pat on the back in the moment when you empty the dishwasher, make a couple of phone calls you've been putting off, get the car washed, or stay at work 20 minutes later than usual to finish up a task. Or do a mental accounting while taking a relaxing bath, enjoying a cup of tea before dinner, or sitting in front of a roaring fire at the end of the day. Or fill out the form on page 159 if that makes your accomplishments more concrete and you like writing things down. **Do not use the form at all on your worst days until you have done it a dozen times when you feel relatively good about what you've gotten done.** The idea is to get attuned to noticing what you've gotten done.

DISARMING YOUR SAD NEMESIS: STRESS MANAGEMENT

↗ FAST FACTS

- Stress is a mental, physical, and emotional phenomenon—it cuts into your ability to think, act, and regulate emotion.

- Some things are stressful for everyone (a loved one's illness, financial difficulties, etc.), but other stresses are specific to the individual: know yourself.

- Summer is the time to plan how to minimize winter stress.

- Getting more done in the summer than you typically do will ease winter pressure to do more than you can.

Stress is part of everyone's life. Sometimes it's positive—the stress of competition that pushes you to some new achievement that you value—and some stresses in our lives are unavoidable even when they're negative. But there's a lot you can do to manage the rest of the stressors in your life, and when you have SAD, doing so is one of the most powerful tools you have.

Most of us know—or think we know—what causes us the most damaging stress in our lives. But a quick survey can help uncover hidden sources of stress that you can wrestle to the mat:

Be Aware

What types of events/activities do you anticipate with dread or worry?

_____

_____

My Accomplishments for the Day

Be Aware

List your accomplishments (including those that seem minor or inconsequential, such as getting out of bed when you planned to and making yourself a sandwich for lunch) and then rate on a scale of 1–10 how getting that task affected your mood, from 1 for not at all to 10 for great improvement.

If you like, you can use how your mood responded to getting something done to plan what to do tomorrow and also what skills you learned from getting these tasks done.

Date: _____

Accomplishments:

_____

_____

_____

_____

_____

_____

Change in mood afterward:

_____

_____

_____

_____

_____

_____

Based on how my accomplishments affected my mood, tomorrow I will try my best to do:

_____

_____

_____

_____

_____

_____

New skills I learned:

_____

_____

What types of events/activities leave you feeling most exhausted?

_____

_____

What kinds of thoughts keep you up at night?

_____

_____

What types of thoughts keep you in bed in the morning?

_____

_____

What types of events/activities make you feel refreshed and energized?

_____

_____

What types of events/activities make you feel relaxed and happy?

_____

_____

Melissa loved old movies, which she tended to start late in the evening, going to bed after midnight and then having even more trouble getting up in the morning than SAD itself caused. When she finally yanked herself out of bed, she already felt guilty about "ruining the day" and started ruminating about all that she wouldn't get done.

What could she do to spare herself this predictable consequence?

_____

_____

Jonathan had served on the hospital board for years and felt good about the contribution he made to, and the respect he got from, the community for this service.

But the meetings were long and sometimes contentious, and more and more often they left him drained for a week.

What could he do to avoid this exhaustion?

_____

_____

Sasha thought she was a terrible mother. The minute the holiday decorations came down, SAD kept her from doing most of the things she wanted to do with her kids for fun. Sometimes she felt she barely took care of their fundamental needs before collapsing into bed at night.

How could she explain to a 2- and 4-year-old that Mommy couldn't do the same things with them in the winter that she did all the time in the warmer seasons?

_____

_____

These may seem like mundane problems with obvious solutions. But stress is a balancing act that always requires weighing the positives and negatives. If Melissa gave up her movies altogether, she'd miss out on a nondemanding source of pleasure in the darkest months when she had little energy to go very far afield. She decided to save the movies for weekend afternoons and switched to watching TV series she'd missed, sticking to a 1-hour episode every night. She could also check out Chapter 13 to help her identify other pleasant activities to add to her daily or weekly routine.

Stress Lesson 1

Looking at our life situations as all black or white can lead to denying ourselves pleasure while ridding ourselves of pain. Always seek the compromise that preserves the positives.

Jonathan couldn't bear to resign from the board. The fact that the younger directors relied on him and his grasp of the board's history made him feel obligated to stay. He also derived some satisfaction from feeling needed. So, instead of continuing to worry about what would happen if he left (worry that was upsetting his stomach on a regular basis), he and another senior director hashed out a plan to train other board members to take over some of his duties, to put a time limit on the agenda (the threat of having to meet again over the weekend if they didn't address the whole agenda in the time allowed had a remarkable effect in smoothing discussion and planning), and to retire the following year but stay on as a consultant. Knowing that he could continue in a less demanding role was a great relief for Jonathan.

Stress Lesson 2

Prepare When we're under stress, it's often our thoughts about an activity or event—forecasting or rehashing—that are the source of stress, and a little strategic planning can ease the present. Depression makes events and activities seem more stressful, and breaking them down into component parts can reduce that stress.

Sasha can probably make some of the effects of SAD understandable to even her very young children ("You know how we all get tired when it gets dark, because it's bedtime? Well, it gets dark a lot earlier now than it does when it's warm outside, and this makes me more tired"), but that may not make the kids miss playtime with her any less, and Sasha really doesn't want them to miss out at all. Her husband suggested getting a teenage babysitter to come over and play with them for a couple of hours every afternoon. Sasha had a better idea: She hired a woman to spend that time doing the laundry, starting a good warm dinner, and running errands while she devoted the time to playing with the kids. When she was feeling really SAD, they mainly cuddled on the couch and read together or, in a pinch, watched some TV. When it was sunny, she took advantage of the light and took the kids outdoors to play in the snow. On weekends, she enlisted her husband to alternate between errands/chores and playing with the kids so that the kids got active time with at least one parent every day.

Stress Lesson 3

Don't try to be a superhero. Be realistic about what you can do without stressing yourself to the max and get whatever help you can afford. Recruit those who care about you to lend support and assistance. Sometimes people with SAD need help maintaining a sense of their priorities, so if you feel overwhelmed by trying to choose what to tackle and what you can let go, try talking it through with your partner or a supportive friend. Try not to sacrifice what makes you feel good to meet mundane obligations if you have any other alternative.

Depression has a way of making everything look black and white (mostly on the dark side), and we can get so focused on the goal of eliminating whatever seems to cause us pain that we forget what an essential ingredient pleasure is in any recipe for lowering stress—a point the preceding examples illustrate. Go to Chapters 13 and 14 for help with identifying pleasurable activities and challenging negative thoughts and beliefs. An entire school of thought called "positive psychology" has arisen in the last 20 years that recognizes the importance of taking active steps to make life more fulfilling, not just solve psychological problems. See the Resources at the back of the book if you're interested in reading more about this. We can also forget that we need and deserve the support of others in our life; some ideas for how to get it appear later in this chapter.

Don't Let the (Short) Days Get Away from You

Treat
A lot of stress reduction is really time management. You may already use time management tools and skills at work, and there's no reason you can't extend them to cover the daily hours outside of work as well. You'll find a wealth of terrific tools with a simple Internet search for "time management" (or, for that matter, "stress management"). One site that offers a wide variety of well-researched free tools and techniques is *www.mindtools.com*, which offers apps for your smartphone too. You can use the Daily Mood Log in Chapter 6 to draw connections between your mood and certain stressful or exciting events that occurred if you're already filling out the log on a regular basis. If you're having trouble figuring out your priorities or agonizing over dropping any of your obligations, an alternative to getting someone to help you sort things out is to use the form on page 163 to record how you spend your time. Some people (with and without SAD) find that they learn an awful lot about their priorities by keeping this record for even a few days. *But remember: Forms like these are tools, not homework assignments. If they don't feel like they'll get you closer to your SAD solution, pass them by.*

What can you learn from recording how you spend your time?

- *Exactly how much time you spend on certain routine activities compared to others.* Are you spending more time than you want to or need to on certain activities, putting you in a pinch for other obligations so that you end up irritable and wiped out by evening?

- *How you might shift activities around to schedule them at the best time.* If you can see that you feel groggy and have difficulty concentrating between 9:00 and 11:00 when you make sales calls, can you schedule them at a time when your focus and energy are sharper? If you feel exhausted and pressured trying to get dinner started right after work, can you spend a weekend morning cooking and freezing dishes that you only have to reheat on weeknights? If you're tired after dinner, when the kids are finished with homework and want to spend time with you, can you use the time you're no longer spending on cooking to give them some quality time before dinner?

- *Your priorities.* What can you let drop—or at least drop down to the bottom of your must-do list? Maybe you feel like you *should* make the kids your top priority when you get home from work but you realize that a menial task like folding the laundry or doing yard work when you get home is an important transitional activity where you don't have to think and that also leaves you feeling like your environment is in order—more in control and less stressed.

See if you can log your activities at least once during the winter. Trying to remember how you spent even the most recent days in order to reallocate your time and other resources is likely to be less than successful.

Speaking of memory . . .

TOOLS

Prevent

Tools You Can Use: Electronic Reminders and Calendars

Depression causes problems with concentration and memory, and trying to keep all your appointments and similar information in your head for easy retrieval can cause stress—as can the guilt of missing appointments or arriving late. You may already use Microsoft Outlook or another calendar on your computer, but if you don't, now is a good time to start. Many calendars not only keep track of appointments but also issue reminders, share plans with groups, keep and organize your contacts, file to-do lists, and send invitations to events.

Many people today do all of this with a single electronic device that they can carry around: a smartphone. New apps for smartphones come on the market every day that can help you keep control of your schedule and lower your stress.

Prevent

Keep a File of Go-To People

No matter how well you organize your time, anticipate low energy, and learn to cut yourself slack when you need it, you can never be sure exactly when and how you'll need help. When you need assistance, you might also find phone numbers or even names eluding you. Therefore many people with SAD compile a file of helpers, organizing their list by what the person can do for them, contact information, and any notes on availability. I recommend that you keep this list in your smartphone or PDA or on your computer—easy to search for what you need and easy to edit.

How I Spend My Time

Enter the date (and day of week because it can help to see the differences between workdays and nonworkdays) and time period of the activity, a description of what you did, how you felt at that time of day (both because of SAD symptoms and as a reaction to the activity), and a rating for how important the activity was *to you*. Its importance or value to you may have something to do with how important it is to someone else (such as finishing a project whose success will influence the job review and potential raise or promotion you get from your boss, or going on a school field trip that your child really wants you to attend), but not necessarily.

Day/time period	Activity/event	Mood/feelings	Importance to me (1–5)

Example:

Babysitters
Mom: 777-888-9999; last-minute every day
Samantha: 111–222–3333; after 3 p.m. on weekdays (not always available)
Aunt Tess: 555–666–0000; weekends, sometimes last-minute
Gerta: 123–456–7890 (the agency); $15 an hour (can get here on her own)

Other categories you might list: accountant, cleaning person, handyman, yard workers, taxi service, pet sitters, dog walkers, and so forth. You might even include a miscellaneous category listed under a capital *H* for "help," because sometimes it's hard to remember names in the middle of winter.

Transcending Stress

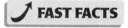

A review of nine controlled studies has shown that regularly practicing transcendental meditation (TM) lowers blood pressure—both while meditating and afterward. High blood pressure is a so-called silent killer and a dangerously common byproduct of excess stress. TM can instill all-day tranquility in practitioners, which means their stress response has been lowered—and that, for SAD sufferers, means less acute depression symptoms and less pressure to get things done during a season marked by low energy. Turn to Chapter 12 for more on TM and other types of meditation.

GETTING SUPPORT

FAST FACTS

- Support can be as simple as having a close confidant or two or as formal as joining an established support group.

- A friend or relative may be willing to offer support for your anti-SAD efforts in exchange for something completely different that you feel able to provide, whereas in a group you may be expected to provide mutual support for experiences related directly to seasonality.

- SAD and other depression-focused support organizations are listed in the Resources at the back of the book.

- If you have difficulty finding support in your community, you may feel motivated to start a group to help others once your own symptoms have eased significantly.

As people with other "invisible" illnesses have found, understanding, compassion, and help can be hard to come by without a few caring individuals in your corner. If you have SAD, I hope you can count on the support of family members and can enlist the aid of some trusted friends, especially when you need to push on through a tough winter. People who offer true support can:

- Provide understanding and promote your own acceptance of the disorder.

- Provide companionship without demands when you don't have much to give.

- Remind you when your acceptance is low that the seasons pass, and this one will pass too.

- Gently encourage you to do what you're trying to do to help yourself (the key word being *gently*).

- Quietly take on some of your chores or other responsibilities in winter without taking your dignity along with them.

How do you ask for support from someone who has not yet learned that you have SAD or milder seasonality? Honesty is the best policy, and education is the best route to support. Offer family or friends a copy of this book or of *Winter Blues* if they want to learn about all aspects of the disorder. Or print out a copy of the handout in the appendix to give to people who need a briefer summary.

Before telling any individual about your seasonal problem, think about what kind of support you would like to receive from that person. Sometimes all you want is understanding for the fact that you will behave differently in the winter than in the summer so that you don't have to apologize for your limitations every winter. With some people you might hope for a sounding board—a confidant you can count on to listen empathically. With others you may be hoping for active assistance. If so, try to think ahead about what kind of help you feel comfortable asking for from that person so you don't leave those who care about you uncertain about what would help and unsure whether they should ask or so that *you* don't hesitate to ask because you're afraid of imposing.

It's also important to keep in mind that friends and family may feel neglected during your SAD season because you might have trouble reaching out to them as you do at other times of year. Intimate partners and spouses may feel physically neglected due to the lack of libido in those with SAD during winter. Knowing ahead of time that your withdrawal is nothing personal may ease any hurt felt by those you care about, as will making up for the lack of attention when your springtime energy returns. Still, you might be careful about what you ask from whom, because if your request is denied, you might end up feeling worse.

**Be
Aware**

How Would You Like People to Support You?

☐ Understand what SAD is and how it affects me.

☐ Spend time with me even if I can't contribute much.

☐ Remind me that this season will pass and that I have more to offer at other times of year and will again.

☐ Help me with little things that are a big hassle for me at my low time of year:

   ☐ Bring me a precooked meal occasionally.

   ☐ Babysit.

   ☐ Run an errand for me.

   ☐ Call me on the phone even though I might not hold up my end of the conversation.

   ☐ Come visit me and help or just chat with me while I do chores.

   ☐ Help me with laundry or housecleaning.

   ☐ Take me to a movie or out for coffee.

   ☐ Go on a winter vacation with me.

☐ Help me even when I don't seem to need it, in spring or summer, if I get too manic and don't remember that this is part of SAD too.

☐ Be patient with me and try not to criticize me even if I'm hard to be around.

☐ Remember that my behavior around you is not directed *at* you—it's nothing personal.

☐ Reject the temptation to try to make me feel fine (we'll both feel better if you don't feel like a failure for not being able to "fix" me).

Don't Forget the Kids!

It's only natural for adults to feel protective of their children, but many people who have SAD have found that explaining what's going on and enlisting some small assistance from even young children makes children feel better than being in the dark and wondering why Mom or Dad is acting so differently these days. In one family I know the whole clan collaborated on a plan to rotate chores, and it was the kids who decided that Mom should be spared bathroom cleaning, the job they all agreed was the worst, during the winter. Wanting and learning how to help is an important aspect of competence that you can nurture in your own children, who will benefit from this capacity as they mature.

Support Groups

SADly, there is only one long-lived major association formed for the exclusive purpose of supporting those with SAD and promoting advances in treatment, and that is the Seasonal Affective Disorder Association based in the United Kingdom. The website is, of course, accessible no matter where you live, and the association can provide lots of material that you might find helpful. But if you want to meet with a group in person to share experiences and ideas, you may have to form one yourself.

Is this something you can ask one of your individual supporters to help with? Maybe you can find an Internet-savvy friend who will set up a chat room or forum for you.

Meanwhile, refer to the list of support-providing organizations in the Resources at the back of this book and check their websites often. This is a great way to keep abreast of advances in research and treatment as they unfold.

☀ *Someone to Talk To*

For some people, the fear of burdening others with their problems adds stress rather than promising support. With acceptance I hope you'll feel more comfortable talking to others about SAD, but if that time has not come, having someone to talk to who understands the problem and can offer empathy and advice is a good reason to seek professional help. Therapists, counselors, and even clergy members may prove to be good (and confidential) outlets for you. It may be hard to put together a support group, but much easier to find one or two people with SAD with whom you can e-mail, share stories, and exchange SAD solution ideas.

WHAT HAVE YOU LEARNED ABOUT ACCEPTANCE, STRESS MANAGEMENT, AND SUPPORT?

Sometimes writing down what you gained (or where your expectations weren't met) helps gel your thoughts and stimulate new ideas. If you think it might help you plan for next year, jot down a few notes about how you'll continue to use the tools in this chapter to gradually increase your level of acceptance, prevent and manage stress, and get the support you need.

_____

_____

_____

Adding this information to your action plan in Chapter 6 can keep it useful as an up-to-date reference.

10

A Life(style) Less SAD

Exercise, Supplements, and Substances

For *at least a third* of those with SAD, light therapy alone is not enough to alleviate symptoms. Stress management definitely helps, but reducing stress is often a gradual process. Fortunately, you have many other self-help tools at your disposal. The strategies in this chapter and the next one can be woven fairly seamlessly into your daily life, they have proven benefits for mood, and as a bonus they contribute to stress reduction by giving your overall health a boost year-round.

WHAT DO YOU HOPE TO GET OUT OF LIFESTYLE CHANGES?

☐ I'm tired of gaining weight every winter and then spending the time of year when I usually feel my best on something that makes me feel worse: dieting.

☐ I want my body to feel better—not constantly achy, stiff, sore, and easily worn out.

☐ I'd like to feel healthier year-round.

☐ I'd like to find additional ways to reduce stress.

CULTIVATE SMALL WINS

The idea of making "lifestyle changes" can sound pretty daunting—making even more effort to get through the day and possibly denying yourself parts of your routine that feel pleasurable or soothing. There's no denying that starting to exercise or eat differently can seem tough at first, but this chapter and Chapter 11 describe how to incorporate these changes gradually and easily so that you can give them a chance to prove how much better they can make you feel. Your goal should be to cultivate small wins. Research has shown that people who make little gains are encouraged to proceed to make bigger gains. *Any* gain is a win, whether it's a few pounds lost, a pair of pants that fits better than before, or being able to run up a flight of stairs without getting winded. Each small win adds up to greater resilience and protection from the "slings and arrows" of daily life so that you can cope better with whatever comes along when your energies are at their lowest due to the season.

You'll get the greatest health and SAD-busting benefits from using the strategies in Chapters 10 and 11 together, but small wins might be easiest if you pick ideas from one chapter or the other to try first. Why not skim both chapters and zero in on the ideas that immediately seem easiest and most appealing? Small wins pile up fastest when you invest your energy where you're most likely to succeed. We discuss exercise before diet simply because exercise can produce some pretty rapid benefits and therefore tends to be self-motivating.

Exercise has great potential for producing small wins, because it offers multiple benefits:

- *Exercise is a proven antidepressant.*

- *Exercise promotes weight control.* Gaining weight due to SAD adds not just pounds but also stress and lowers mood by making you feel worse about yourself.

- *You can exercise outdoors in the early-morning sun for an extra dose of mood-lifting light.*

↗ FAST FACTS

- People with SAD may have slower metabolisms than others.
- Even 20 minutes of exercise a day has health and mood benefits.
- It's important to choose a form of exercise that you enjoy, so you'll stick with it and so it doesn't add to your stress level.

EXERCISE

We all know that exercise is good for us: it tones and builds muscles, promotes cardiovascular health, improves balance and coordination (increasingly critical as we age), burns calories, and helps us sleep better. What may not be as widely known is that exercise is also a proven antidepressant. More and more research shows that exercise improves mood in people with all kinds of depression, including SAD.

An exercise buddy can help you stick with an exercise routine, make the exercise a pleasant activity, provide support, and keep you from withdrawing in the winter

This is great news on paper. But as those suffering SAD know all too well, the fact that something is good for us doesn't necessarily make it easy to implement. Luckily, it doesn't take a lot of experience with exercise to prove the benefits to yourself. You've probably heard workout enthusiasts talk about how bad they feel when they skip their usual routine or how "addicted" they are to the way exercise makes them feel. They may be referring to the pleasant loosening of tight muscles or the fact that it feels good to be physically tired instead of just mentally exhausted. Or they might be referring to the release of soothing endorphins, which have been said to be responsible for the sought-after "runner's high" and may be instrumental in the lift in mood associated with exercise. Hold on to that promise and do whatever you can to get some exercise in the winter.

Make It Fun

The last thing you need is more obligations that feel unpleasant (if you haven't read Chapter 9 yet, now would be a good time to do so). When it's hard to get out of bed, it's even harder to exert the effort to *make* the bed. So realistically, the only way you're likely to give exercise a chance is if it's going to be pleasant. In Chapter 13, you'll find a worksheet that will help you identify activities you enjoy so you can add more of them to your life. There are also many pleasant activity lists available on the Internet. One well-known one contains 140 items. Out of those, roughly 30 (more than 20%) are active pursuits like sports, outdoor recreation, dancing, and walking or hiking. A lot more could involve vigorous exercise, depending on how you do them and for how long.

Chapter 13 and Internet lists can give you a lot of ideas, but to figure out what type of exercise will be fun specifically for *you,* answer the following questions.

☐ Do you find everything more fun if you're doing it with someone you like?

☐ Is it more peaceful (or less stressful, without obligations to socialize) for you to do something active alone, so you can concentrate on thinking pleasant thoughts?

☐ Are you energized by music and lots of activity around you?

☐ Does the beauty of the natural world inspire you?

☐ Does creating or constructing something make exertion feel worthwhile?

☐ Does getting other work done make it easier for you to exercise?

☐ Does competition spur you on?

☐ Do you do your best work when there's a reward waiting for you at the end?

☐ Are you a "Let's get this over with" person or a "I'll tackle this a little at a time" person?

☐ Do you prefer routine or spontaneity?

☐ Do you like games?

What types of exercise your answers lead to is fairly obvious.

If you find the natural environment gives you a lift: Exercise outdoors. This is a particularly potent solution for people with SAD, because it combines exercise with exposure to sunlight, contact with neighbors, and a connection to nature and the seasons. Outdoor exercise ideas are listed on page 174.

If you thrive in the bustle of sounds and activity: Work out at a health club. An added benefit is the support you can get from others pursuing better health, just like you. And the encouragement of a trainer can help you stick with it when you don't feel like it.

If you need company to make things pleasant: Get an exercise buddy or a walking companion. People with SAD often become isolated during winter, and getting your workouts with others can boost your mood through social contact as well as aerobic benefits.

If you've always liked to dance: Take an aerobic dance or Zumba or U-Jam class or go learn salsa or ballroom dancing.

If competition stimulates you: Join a sports team. In our fitness-focused age, many communities have leagues that engage in everything from softball to dodgeball,

Small Wins: Exercise

Every time you achieve a small win from exercising, write it down here. Be specific: A win can be a gain in workouts themselves—extra weight you can lift, greater distance you can run, more laps you can swim, etc.—or the consequence of exercising (a certain number of pounds lost, more energy throughout the day, better sleep, glowing skin, being happier with how you look in the mirror).

_____   _____

_____   _____

_____   _____

_____   _____

_____   _____

If you haven't exercised regularly in the winter (or summer), how can you add it to your routine?

_____

_____

What could you do to add light to your exercise routine?

_____

_____

basketball to jai alai—and there are teams for different age groups. You get the added bonus of company during the matches and at postgame get-togethers.

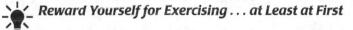 ***Reward Yourself for Exercising . . . at Least at First***

New habits are hard to form for everyone. For those with SAD, getting moving can be doubly difficult. Find a reward that will give you something to look forward to after your workout:

- Give yourself modest shopping trips for a week's workouts or a sojourn in the spa or a massage after your workout.

- Go out for coffee with your workout buddy after you exercise.

- Buy workout clothes that make you feel limber and comfortable.

- Find a new, fun workout to add to your routine: Exercise quickly becomes its own reward, so keep it up and keep it fun.

Treat

Getting More for Your Effort: Exercise Plus Light

Remember, *synergy produces energy.* You can get more bang for your exercise "buck" if you work out in bright light. We don't know whether you'll get greater weight-loss or other benefits from the combination of light and exercise than from exercise alone. We do have some research evidence, however, that light plus exercise has a more potent antidepressant effect than exercise alone, and when you're feeling better you're more likely to stick with the exercise. Obviously, it's pretty easy to get light and exercise at the same time:

- Work out on a treadmill, exercise bike, or other exercise equipment while you get your morning light therapy in front of a light box that has an adjustable-height stand.

- Walk or jog early in the morning in a place where you're exposed to the rising sun.

- Find a health club or gym with machines in front of a window where bright morning light streams through and exercise there.

- Find an indoor pool inside a glass dome and swim laps.

- See if you can find an aerobic fitness class with bright light or that actually has light therapy fixtures. Or suggest to the instructor or business owner that they add them.

- If you enjoy strenuous yard work or even gardening, do it early on sunny days as much as possible.

- Many yoga and Tai Chi classes are held outdoors as the sun rises.

- Outdoor winter sports give you an opportunity to take advantage of direct sunlight and also the reflection of sunlight off the snow and ice.

- Dance studios tend to be brightly lit, which is beneficial even if the light is not at therapeutic levels.

Regular Aerobic Exercise Is Helpful for Summer SAD Too

The antidepressant effects of exercise occur in all the seasons. However, if you have summer SAD and are aware that you feel more agitated or more depressed when exposed to direct, intense summer sunlight, you might want to do your exercising indoors. One woman I know found that swimming in the cold, dark waters of a deep lake was very soothing and therapeutic.

ADDITION AND SUBTRACTION

Regular exercise has a way of increasing your awareness of how your body feels. Becoming more coordinated, energetic, lithe, and agile can make every day easier. With heightened awareness of your physical state throughout the day, you might also find that you're more conscious of your mental, physical, and emotional response to other stimuli in your environment and other things you ingest. This may be why fitness enthusiasts often start to think twice about whether to use alcohol, drugs, tobacco, and even caffeine and also whether they have any dietary deficiencies that could be corrected with supplements. Being even slightly hung over can ruin a workout. Smoking certainly affects your lung power. Being deficient in certain vitamins can leave you vulnerable to viruses. Naturally, diet plays a big role in how you feel as well, and we'll get to that larger subject in the next chapter. For now, you might want to consider what you could add or subtract from your daily routine to feel healthier overall, particularly those substances and supplements that have an impact on SAD symptoms.

Supplements for SAD

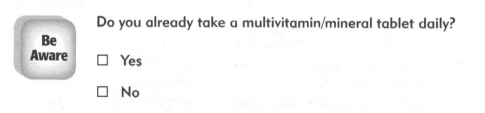

Do you already take a multivitamin/mineral tablet daily?

☐ **Yes**

☐ **No**

Are there other supplements you should consider?

If you don't already take a daily vitamin, now is a good time to start. Ask your doctor whether, based on your overall health profile, there is a particular combination or strength you should be looking for. Otherwise, there is a huge variety of options available today, for men and women, for people over age 50, for pregnant/

lactating women, and so forth. Depending on your daily food intake to supply all the vitamins and minerals you need is iffy.

⫰⫰⫰ SCIENCE

In a study of almost 15,000 older male doctors over more than 10 years, those who took a daily multivitamin instead of a placebo were found to have 8% fewer cancers. The study, completed in 2012, was one of the largest and longest studies of vitamin use. SAD aside, taking a multivitamin pill every day seems to make sense.

Vitamin D

Although there is some debate over how many of us need a supplement and at what dosage, we do know most of us are deficient in vitamin D, partly because we all use sunscreen these days and possibly also because many adults don't consume a lot of vitamin-D-enriched milk. Vitamin D is synthesized through the skin from the sun's UV rays, and we can't give up our sunblock and go back to risking skin cancer. So how do you know whether you need vitamin D supplements?

- ☐ **Are you at risk otherwise for the conditions from which vitamin D protects us? (See the box on page 177.)**

- ☐ **Do you live in the North?**

- ☐ **Has a blood test shown a deficiency?**

- ☐ **Does your doctor recommend it?**

If you're reading this book, of course there is a good chance you live in the North and need help with SAD symptoms. Ironically, all the efforts you may make to get outdoors in the sun to increase your exposure to light may not bump up your vitamin D levels, again because you're using necessary sunscreen.

The question uppermost in your mind might be whether vitamin D has any beneficial effects on SAD itself. Some individuals with SAD have reported improved mood after starting vitamin D_3 (the active form of the vitamin), but so far there are no controlled studies (those in which the group taking the substance, in this case vitamin D, is compared with a group not taking it) to back this up. Still, with vitamin D contributing to cardiac health and other important functions, it's good to know whether you have a deficiency. A reliable test called 25-OH Vitamin D can detect a deficiency, which can be corrected with the proper dosage in supplements.

Why We Need Vitamin D

Be Aware

- As we've always been told, vitamin D helps build and maintain strong bones.

- It *might* help prevent cancer, dementia, diabetes, some autoimmune diseases, and heart disease.

- It might promote muscle strength, which may be why it has been seen to prevent the falls (and fractures) common among older people.

- It boosts immunity.

- It reduces inflammation.

When the data are analyzed in 2016 from an NIH study of 20,000 adults, we should have a better idea of whether vitamin D really does prevent cancer and cardiovascular disease.

Because vitamin D is a fat-soluble vitamin and stored longer than water-soluble vitamins like C and B, it's important not to take too much. Consult your doctor or physician's assistant.

Other Supplements for SAD

Treat

You may be interested in trying B vitamins, which have shown some benefits for depression:

- ☑ Vitamin B$_1$ (thiamine): 50 mg a day elevated mood in four different controlled studies.

- ☑ Vitamin B$_{12}$ and Folic acid: There are no clear guidelines for exactly what dosage will help with depression, but a good place to start is with a standard B complex supplement.

- ☑ Fish oil (omega-3 fatty acids): 1–2 grams a day. Most people take fish oil for its heart-health benefits, but it *might* help both depression and bipolar disorder, though research evidence has been mixed. Flax seed oil is a decent substitute for vegetarians.

☑ **St. John's wort:** The evidence that this herbal extract is an effective anti-depressant is abundant enough, but sadly it also makes those who take it sensitive to sunlight, increasing the risk for sunburn or eye pain. Because of reports of eye pain when taking St. John's wort and using light therapy (although they are only anecdotal), I don't recommend St. John's wort for those using light therapy at the same time. If you decide to try it because you are not using a light box, know that it can also cause sexual and sleep problems as well as irritability (though these are often less marked than with antidepressant medications).

Substances and SAD

And now for the subtractions: Many people believe that a couple of cocktails or glasses of wine really improves their mood. And alcohol might do that, at least temporarily. But that boost probably won't be worth it, because alcoholic beverages are likely to rob you of energy and send your mood further downward for a few days afterward. In fact, what you drink on Saturday night might not cause a rebound depression until *two* days afterward, which can make it hard to connect your weekend activity with your weekday mood.

Exercise even more caution where marijuana is concerned. Marijuana may at first make you feel mildly blissful, but at the cost of a cluster of symptoms that only makes SAD worse: increased depression, lethargy, and lack of motivation. In addition, it can be addictive. Finally, marijuana is notorious for causing people to snack with abandon—the last thing you need if it lowers your inhibitions and leads you to obey any carb cravings.

Treat

What could you do (particularly in the evening) to relax in place of using alcohol or marijuana?

☐ Have a cup of tea

☐ Take an evening walk

☐ Take a warm bath with fragrant candles

☐ Read enjoyable books or poetry

☐ Listen to soothing or uplifting music

☐ Call a friend

☐ Meet a friend for a walk or dinner

☐ Meditate

☐ Do relaxation exercises (see Chapter 12)

☐ Go to a movie, play, or concert

Small Wins: Substituting for Substances

Record here anytime you replace use of alcohol or marijuana with some other, healthier (and actually effective) remedy for the blues:

_____   _____

_____   _____

_____   _____

_____   _____

WHAT HAVE YOU LEARNED ABOUT EXERCISE, SUPPLEMENTS, AND SUBSTANCES?

Sometimes writing down what you gained (or where your expectations weren't met) helps gel your thoughts and stimulate new ideas. If you think it might help you plan for next year, jot down a few thoughts about how you might add exercise, take advantage of supplements, and subtract substances.

_____

_____

_____

What routes would you like to try to control your weight?

☐ **Exercise: Start small so you get those little wins, but try to start soon!**

☐ **Diet: Turn to the next chapter.**

☐ **Stress management: See Chapter 9.**

☐ **Meditation: See Chapter 12.**

Adding this information to your action plan in Chapter 6 can keep it useful as an up-to-date reference.

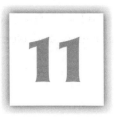

11

Dietary Strategies
for Controlling Weight
and SAD

★ KEY POINTS

For many people with SAD, one of the toughest effects of seasonality is weight gain. Fortunately, awareness of what causes winter weight gain provides you with a wealth of ideas, collected in this chapter, for keeping weight under control.

For a variety of SAD-related reasons, seasonal depression can make us eat more and exercise less. The result is too many calories going in and too few going out. Some of the weight gained in winter* may come off starting in spring, but in many cases extra pounds are retained. Not only does excess weight contribute to a long list of health problems, but it's a morale buster that only makes depression worse. As explained earlier in this book, you may crave sugary, starchy foods because for many people with SAD they seem to boost serotonin levels and, with them, mood. So that bag of cookies holds a lot of immediate gratification when you're really down. Unfortunately, it holds the promise of a lot of weight gain, especially because those with SAD may burn off the calories more slowly than nonseasonal people (see the facing page).

Controlling your weight may not seem easy if you've gained weight winter after winter, especially if you've found losing the extra pounds in summer increasingly difficult over the years. As with the rest of your SAD solution, success starts

---

*People with summer SAD tend to have reduced appetite and may lose weight rather than gain it.

with awareness. When you know what foods and behaviors tend to pack on the pounds, and what your patterns of eating and weight gain have been, you're armed to fight the battle of the bulge.

↗ FAST FACTS

- High-glycemic-index foods—those that quickly dump carbohydrates into the bloodstream (candy, for example)—give you a quick boost in energy and mood and then a correspondingly deep crash in blood sugar, creating the urge to eat again right away.

- Many people gain a little weight in the winter. People with SAD tend to gain a lot more.

- Winter weight gains become harder and harder to shed over the years.

- Yielding to carb cravings can, over time, lead to diabetes.

- Diets lower in carbohydrates and higher in lean protein (fish, for example) and low-glycemic-index, complex carbs (such as legumes) preserve energy, protect health, and help prevent weight gain.

Even a challenge like weight control is manageable when you break it down into steps. Following are four straightforward steps that can help you maintain a healthy body weight throughout the year.

Be Aware WEIGHT CONTROL STEP 1: UNDERSTAND WHAT CONTRIBUTES TO WEIGHT GAIN AND HOW *YOUR* EATING AND WEIGHT ARE CONNECTED

🧪 SCIENCE

People with SAD may have a slower metabolism than others, according to one study by a Siberian researcher. If that's the case for you, and you're trying to lose weight, *aerobic exercise* could be your friend: it not only burns calories but increases metabolism after you finish working out. But *weight training* is a friend too: muscle cells burn calories faster than fat cells.

By how many pounds does your weight fluctuate during the year?

☐ 0–3   ☐ 4–7   ☐ 8–11   ☐ 12–15   ☐ 16–20   ☐ Over 20

Do your food preferences change from season to season?

☐ No   ☐ Yes

How?

_____

_____

_____

The more weight you gain in the winter, the more important it may be for you to consider measures to manage your diet. (If you have summer SAD, you're more likely to eat less and to lose weight during your problematic season, so the advice in this section applies only to winter SAD. We have no evidence that any dietary changes are helpful in summer SAD.) So-called yo-yo dieting—gaining and losing repeatedly—is linked with heart disease and other health problems, and the longer you yo-yo, the harder it becomes to lose the weight each year. In addition, of course, gaining a lot of weight can be demoralizing, adding to depression and stress.

 Some people with SAD struggle to keep their weight under control year-round, although most eat more than they would like and gain the most weight in winter. Many people who are not overweight love sweets and starches, so how do you tell if you are a true carb craver? Do any of these behaviors sound familiar?

☐ **When you feel like you need a snack, do you reach for cookies, cake, crackers, cereal, bread, or even fruit and fruit juices instead of celery sticks or nuts?**

☐ **Do you ever grab a bag of chips or pretzels with the intention of having a few and then end up shocked that you've gone through the whole bag without noticing what you were doing?**

☐ **If you eat a bagel or a bowl of cereal with fruit at 8:00 A.M., do you find yourself hungrier at 10:00 than if you had eaten a hard-boiled egg or nothing at all?**

☐ **If you want seconds at dinner, do you usually have more bread or potatoes instead of more salad or protein?**

☐ Do you eat high-carbohydrate snacks between meals or after dinner most days of the week?

☐ Does overindulgence in cookies or chips or the like perk you up, at least briefly?

The more items you checked, the more likely you are a carb craver and would benefit from managing what you eat, especially during the winter if that's when you tend to gain the most weight. For most people, the consequence of eating a lot of the carbs that we used to call "quick sugars" is weight gain. For those of us with SAD, the end result is often even greater weight gain, but also a roller-coaster mood ride between highs and lows—up and energized with sugar intake, down and lethargic with the quick drops in blood sugar that follow.

⚗ SCIENCE

Metabolic Syndrome

Metabolic syndrome is a collection of health problems that raise the risk of type 2 diabetes, stroke, and coronary artery disease. If you have three or more of the following signs, you can reduce that risk with lifestyle changes like managing your diet and exercising.

☐ High blood pressure

☐ High blood sugar

☐ Low HDL cholesterol

☐ High triglycerides

☐ Large waist

Having SAD can contribute to the development of metabolic syndrome by causing you to increase your sugar intake, gain weight, and decrease exercise. Your physician can tell you whether you're in the danger zone for any of these signs. *If you are, don't panic. Just start taking a slow and gentle approach to making changes, according to your doctor's advice, in lifestyle areas like diet and activity level.*

⚠ **Carbohydrates, especially the "bad" ones—quick sugars or simple carbs—actually increase hunger, causing overeating, instead of satisfying it.**

HOW CARBOHYDRATES END UP BEING
BAD FOR US

Here's how the consumption of carbohydrates works:

1. I eat a cookie.

2. The sugar in the cookie enters the bloodstream (resulting in a rise of what we call "blood sugar"). I'm not really hungry anymore.

3. The pancreas recognizes the sugar in the bloodstream and sends insulin to push the sugar into the body tissues, such as fat, lowering blood sugar.

4. The drop in blood sugar triggers hunger.

5. I eat another cookie. Or three.

Actual sugar, as in the kind in a cookie, enters and leaves the bloodstream quickly (which is why it is known as a "quick sugar"), and the precipitous drop in blood sugar makes us hungry soon after eating. The upshot? We eat more and we do so more often.

Now let's add SAD to the picture:

1. I eat a cookie.

2. The sugar enters the bloodstream. I'm not really hungry anymore.

3. The pancreas secretes insulin to move the sugar along. Meanwhile, insulin also moves tryptophan into the brain, where that amino acid is the building block for serotonin production.

4. I feel a lot less depressed.

5. But then my blood sugar drops precipitously—perhaps even more precipitously than for my nonseasonal neighbor who ate the same cookie, because research shows that people with SAD secrete more insulin, meaning my blood sugar drops lower once the insulin has done its transportation work.

6. I eat three more cookies very soon, because I'm really hungry again while my neighbor is still satiated.

The upshot? Because I have SAD, not only do foods packed with simple carbs, like cookies, provide a desperately needed (but short-lived) mood boost, but my overeager insulin secretion makes me need a premature refill. I gain even more weight than my nonseasonal neighbor, and I may be more prone to metabolic syndrome. The fat that builds up from my carb bingeing, especially the fat around the belly, is more resistant to insulin, which means the pancreas has to work harder and harder to secrete more and more insulin over time. Eventually the pancreas stops secreting as much insulin as is needed, and blood sugar builds—my blood tests begin to show high blood sugar and, if the cycle continues, the end result is diabetes.

The solution?

WEIGHT CONTROL STEP 2: CUT DOWN ON SIMPLE CARBS

Now that you have a grasp of the fundamentals of weight gain, it's fairly easy to see that cutting down on high-impact (weight-increasing) carbohydrates is a good first step to avoiding weight gain this year . . . and every year.

> To prevent weight gain in the winter that might still be with you in the summer, don't try to starve yourself; focus on your choice of foods instead.

Tools You Can Use: The Glycemic Index

The glycemic index (GI) is a measure of how quickly various foods you eat will release sugar into your bloodstream. It was originated at the University of Toronto in the early 1980s by doctors who were trying to determine which types of food were healthiest for those with diabetes. The index lists foods on a scale of 1–100, with pure glucose having a glycemic index of 100. Glycemic index ratings for a given food that you eat may vary based on how much you eat, what your blood sugar was when you started eating, whether you've already developed insulin resistance as described on the facing page, and the condition (ripeness, freshness, and form) of the food eaten. Nutritionists warn against using the GI rating as the sole measure of whether a food will be "good for you," and it may be wise to use it mainly as a guide for comparing foods usually considered rich in carbs—fruits, starchy vegetables, grains, sugars, breads, pastas, and the like. The index is a good measure of where a food stands between the simplest of simple carbs on the weight-adding end and the most complex of complex carbs on the weight-controlling end of the cornucopia of foods available to us.

Basically, the more fiber a carbohydrate has, the more natural its state, and the less sweet it tastes, the lower the GI.

If a food gives you that quick, satisfied feeling or sugar high, chances are you are best off avoiding it. When you learn to monitor your carbohydrate intake, you can become very sensitive to detecting carbohydrate-rich foods. Favor foods that satisfy more slowly. Over time, those foods will become increasingly satisfying, and the high-impact carbs may become less appealing, making you feel too full, too heady, or simply off balance.

⚠ *Avoid White Carbohydrates!*

White sugar, white bread, pasta, white rice—all of these foods have a higher GI than their deeper-colored counterparts.

Much more comprehensive lists of foods by GI are available online (search "glycemic index food list"), but here are some ideas for what you might substitute:

Instead of . . .	Try . . .
Cornflakes or Rice Krispies	Oatmeal,* oat bran, or muesli
French fries	Sweet potato
Bagel	Whole-grain toast
Pretzels	Peanuts
Peas	Green beans
Raisins (calories densely packed)	Cherries (calories less densely packed)
Soft drinks**	Water or skim milk
Couscous	Beans
Melon	Grapefruit

*Try Irish steel-cut oats in particular; they have a GI of 42 compared to 66 for quick oats!

**Sugary soft drinks, with glucose or high-fructose corn syrup that enters the bloodstream extra rapidly without fiber to slow it down, is especially bad, but artificially sweetened soft drinks may also cause weight gain by tricking the brain into thinking sugar has been consumed and behaving accordingly.

Over time, many people find choosing foods that raise blood sugar slowly becomes intuitive. But you can start by thinking about how you might shift your standard meal choices:

☐ Can you substitute yogurt with whole-grain cereal and half a grapefruit or a couple of boiled eggs for a bagel or doughnut for breakfast?

☐ Can you replace your submarine sandwich with a chef's salad full of crisp vegetables?

☐ Can you snack on nuts instead of chips? Fresh fruit like grapes and berries instead of a candy bar?

☐ Can you give up your lattes in favor of regular coffee with skim milk?

☐ Can you serve a whole-wheat tortilla as the bread to go with dinner instead of a baguette?

☐ Can you have fruit and a few nuts instead of pie for dessert?

Small Wins: High-Impact Carbohydrate Consumption

Record any way that you have replaced high-GI foods with low-GI foods. It's okay to include single-meal achievements, but give yourself a resounding cheer when you make these changes a habit:

_____   _____

_____   _____

_____   _____

_____   _____

_____   _____

_____   _____

_____   _____

Treat

WEIGHT CONTROL STEP 3:
EAT LIKE A NEANDERTHAL

Weight control is not just a matter of avoiding high-impact carbohydrates but of substituting foods that are higher in protein and fiber and lower in carbohydrates overall. We're not suggesting you go out and club some wild animal for dinner, but many of the most effective weight-loss diets today emphasize low-carb foods like greens and other vegetables, berries, and moderate amounts of protein—a regimen somewhat like that of the hunter-gatherers of prehistory. The theory is that many modern ills, from heart disease and diabetes to tooth decay, arose along with agriculture. After farming started, we gained access to larger quantities of grains, sources of sugar like corn and beets, and cultivated produce. Then we refined them—and started gaining weight and losing robust health.

Some Ideas for Featuring These Foods

Breakfast:

Eggs or egg substitutes

Oatmeal (not instant) with walnut bits or pepitas

Breakfast burrito wrapped in a whole-wheat tortilla

Protein shakes (check the ingredient label for carbs if store-bought)

Lunch:

Green salad with meat or fish added

Tuna or salmon salad

Vegetable soup (without grains or pasta, which can make soup high in carbs)

Snacks:

Unsalted nuts

Cottage cheese or part-skim mozzarella cheese sticks (string cheese)

Celery sticks and low-fat cheese spread (such as Laughing Cow)

Dinner:

Grilled lean meat or fish

Steamed greens (spinach, chard, kale, cabbage, etc.)

Other steamed green vegetables (broccoli, green beans, asparagus, etc.)

Sautéed mixed greens with mushrooms and a small amount of vegetables containing low-impact carbohydrates (eggplant, broccoli, etc.) with a dash of soy sauce

Stews and soups without starchy vegetables

You'll find a lot more ideas and recipes at websites set up by originators of popular low-carb diets like Atkins, the Zone, Protein Power, Sugar Busters, South Beach, and others:

- *www.atkins.com*
- *www.zonediet.com*
- *www.proteinpower.com*
- *www.sugarbusters.com*
- *www.southbeachdiet.com*

TOOLS

Tools You Can Use: A Scale

Do you hate weighing yourself?

☐ **Yes**

☐ **No**

If the idea of getting on a scale is so repellent to you that it makes you want to avoid thinking about food altogether, perhaps you should avoid weighing yourself because it simply adds too much to your stress. But instead of thinking of your scale as a nag, try to think of it as a tool. If you weigh yourself every day *and write down your weight,* you can gather data about what makes your weight go up when winter arrives and what makes it go down when you're trying to manage your diet and exercise more. You may find that you avoid cravings most when you adhere to a fairly steady low-carb diet or that you're just fine as long as you avoid foods with the highest GI rating. Particular foods may seem irresistible, and as you avoid them and substitute new, low-GI foods, you may find the high-GI foods less and less appealing.

 TOOLS

Tools You Can Use: A Food Log

If you weigh yourself daily and try to link any gain or loss with what you've been eating, you may emerge with some good ideas for modifying your diet to control your weight. But this process can take time. Another way to decide on changes you wish to make in your diet is to record what you eat for a week or two and then examine your current diet against the advice in this chapter. If you decide to take a closer look at what you're eating, I strongly recommend writing down everything you eat. It's just too easy, especially if you're subject to carb cravings that lead to mindless bingeing and grazing, to get an incomplete picture when you merely try to reconstruct your daily consumption from memory. Use the Food Log on the facing page, making as many copies as you need to record your intake for a week or two (or download the form from *www.guilford.com/rosenthal3-forms*). In the "What I Ate/Drank" column, do your best to include portion size (weight, volume, or other measurement).

To get an idea of whether this exercise might be useful to you, take a look at the examples filled out by Stacey on pages 192 and 193. Stacey figured out with a pretty quick review that every time she ate something with a lot of carbs, she was hungry

Small Gains . . . or *Losses!*

Record here any weight loss, drop in clothing size, or even ability to wear slimmer, closer-fitting clothes that you couldn't before:

_____   _____

_____   _____

_____   _____

_____   _____

_____   _____

Food Log

Date: _____

Time	What I ate/drank	Where?	Planned meal or snack? (Y or N)	What I learned

Food Log

Date: Tuesday, November 5, 2013

Time	What I ate/drank	Where?	Planned meal or snack? (Y or N)	What I learned
7:30 A.M.	Sweet roll, 12-ounce latte	Subway	Y	
9:00 A.M.	Small bagel and 2 tablespoons cream cheese, coffee	Office	N	I was hungry again right after getting to work and ate a doughnut when I didn't really want to.
11:30 A.M.	Chicken Caesar salad, iced tea	Restaurant	Y	Tasted good, and I didn't think about food till it was almost time to go home.
4:00 P.M.	Candy bar	On my way back to subway	N	Still hungry on the train. I was so hungry that dinner wasn't ready.
6:00 P.M.	3 ounces cheese and 12 saltines	Living room while watching news	N	
8:00 P.M.	2 servings beef stew, 3 slices French bread, apple	Still in front of TV	Y	I ate more than I planned and wasn't even going to have the bread. But there it was on the counter. I was watching a funny show and didn't even think about it when I went to the kitchen for another helping of stew and 2 slices of bread. I can't believe I was hungry. And I swore I'd have an apple if I was going to eat in the kitchen. I'd already had ___ for dessert.
11:00 P.M.	2 2-inch square brownies	Living room right before bed	N	

Food Log

Date: _____

Time	What I ate/drank	Where?	Planned meal or snack? (Y or N)	What I learned

Food Log

Date: Tuesday, November 5, 2013

Time	What I ate/drank	Where?	Planned meal or snack? (Y or N)	What I learned
7:30 A.M.	Sweet roll, 12-ounce latte	Subway	Y	
9:00 A.M.	Small bagel and 2 tablespoons cream cheese, coffee	Office	N	I was hungry again right after getting to work and ate a doughnut when I didn't really want to.
11:30 A.M.	Chicken Caesar salad, iced tea	Restaurant	Y	Tasted good, and I didn't think about food till it was almost time to go home.
4:00 P.M.	Candy bar	On my way back to subway	N	Still hungry on the train. I was so hungry, but dinner wasn't ready!
6:00 P.M.	3 ounces cheese and 12 saltines	Living room while watching news	N	
8:00 P.M.	2 servings beef stew, 3 slices French bread, apple	Still in front of TV	Y	I ate more than I planned and wasn't even going to have the bread. But there it was on the counter. I was watching a funny show and didn't even think about it when I went back to the kitchen for another helping of stew and 2 more slices of bread. I can't believe I was hungry again! And I swore I'd have an apple if I was going to snack in the evening . . . but I'd already eaten the apple for dessert.
10:00 P.M.	2 2-inch square brownies	Living room right before bed	N	

Food Log

Date: _Saturday, May 24, 2014_

Time	What I ate/drank	Where?	Planned meal or snack? (Y or N)	What I learned
9:00 A.M.	8-oz. fruit cup, hard-boiled egg, coffee	Kitchen	N	Wasn't hungry when I got up; beautiful day, so I went running and ate when I got home.
12:00 P.M.	Vegetable potstickers (3), shrimp stir-fry, white rice, fortune cookie	Restaurant	Y	Had so much fun talking to my friend at lunch that I didn't end up finishing my lunch and took half of the stir-fry and rice home.
2:00 P.M.	Pita chips and hummus, handful of chocolate-covered raisins	Deck while reading	N	Just felt like doing what I wanted—it's the weekend, finally!
8:00 P.M.	Fried calamari, fettuccine Alfredo, 2 slices Italian bread, green salad with balsamic vinaigrette, 3 glasses red wine, lemon sorbetto	Restaurant	Y	My friends had raved about this new restaurant, and by the time we ate I was starving. Next time I'm going out to eat this late I'll make sure I eat a light snack closer to dinner. I probably wouldn't have eaten that much if I had had only 1 or 2 glasses of wine.

again shortly afterward, and she seemed to eat more and more as the day wore on as a result. Noticing that she was hungrier faster after the sweet roll and latte than after the bagel, she resolved to stick to foods with less sugar for her first meal of the day. She also noted that she went about 4 hours without feeling hungry after lunch and vowed to eat more meals and snacks like that. One thing Stacey realized upon reviewing her log was that she hadn't always specified quantities. She knew that she had eaten more than she wanted to at dinner, but when she thought about what she meant by "2 servings" of beef stew, she was chagrined to realize that they were probably 2-cup servings. If she had measured what she served herself, she might have been more likely to skip the second helping. Finally, Stacey reminded herself that she was moving into winter, and that, while it was all the more important to nip overeating in the bud now, it also meant she needed to be kind to herself. She decided that the next day she'd go buy some of the mixed nuts that she really enjoyed to have on hand as a special snack.

Look at how differently Stacey ate in the spring! Stacey noticed that even with some indulgences, she didn't gain any weight and didn't end up bingeing or feeling like she had to eat again soon, probably because she wasn't seeking the same antidepressant effect she needed in fall and winter. Some protein (the egg) and complex carbs (the fruit) served her well in the morning, after an energizing and metabolism-raising run in the bright morning sun. At lunch it was easy to be diverted from eating too much by enjoying the company. Note, however, that once again Stacey did not record the quantities of pita chips and hummus she ate. When she reached for the same snack the next day, she was dismayed to see that she had eaten half of a large bag of chips and half of a 10-ounce tub of hummus—the hummus alone containing 400 calories, more than half of them from fat. The carbs in the chickpeas may have been low impact, but with that many calories and fat the hummus was a pretty rich snack. She had then overindulged at dinner, and upon review she realized that might have been fueled by the three glasses of wine she drank. But again, probably because she wasn't depressed, she wasn't drawn back to the refrigerator for a late-night snack.

☀ *Breakfasts of SAD Champions*

Breakfast sets the dietary tone for the rest of the day. Notice in Stacey's winter food log that having a sweet roll and large latte left her hungry shortly afterward. An egg-white omelet and steel-cut oatmeal would stay with her (and you) longer. Here are a few tips for starting the day off right:

- **Think of every morning as an opportunity to start afresh, and the name of that fresh start is breakfast. Don't dwell on regrets about how you ate yesterday. Today you are born again.**

- Make sure you have the best breakfast foods on hand at all times. You can't expect to eat right if all you have in the kitchen when you wake up is all the "wrong" foods.

- Even cooked breakfast dishes can be made the night before and microwaved to heat them up. Try making an egg-white omelet stuffed with vegetables in the evening and then zapping it when you get up, before you have a chance to reach for the boxed cereal. Likewise steel-cut oatmeal, which can take 30 minutes to cook: Make enough for the week, store it in the fridge, and reheat the day's portion each morning.

- If you have healthy steamed or sautéed vegetables in the fridge, you can stuff them into a whole-wheat tortilla and heat them in the microwave as a breakfast burrito in mere seconds.

WEIGHT CONTROL STEP 4: AVOID STRESS-DRIVEN EATING

Even with all the best-laid plans you've made and followed in the first three weight control steps, your efforts can go awry if stress is ruling your day. Many, many people eat when under stress. It may be that the physical strain sends a signal to the brain that the body and mind need fortification. It may be "nerves"—the urge to do something to keep busy and get your mind off your worries. It may be simply that eating foods that you find pleasurable is soothing and thus reduces your stress. Whatever the reason, if you find yourself giving in to unplanned eating (see your Food Logs) and carb cravings, try extra measures to reduce stress (see Chapter 9).

Treat

Meditate and Lose Weight!

When I first started to meditate, I was amazed to find that I lost 8 pounds without even trying over several months. Because meditation was the only new addition to my regimen, I had to conclude that meditating, by reducing my stress, was reducing my stress-driven eating. Others have seen the same happy result. Turn to Chapter 12 to find out whether you'd like to learn and practice meditation. Also consider reading *The Hunger Fix,* by Pamela Peeke (see the Resources), which stresses the value of dealing with stress and specifically mentions the use of meditation as one valuable technique.

Whether you recorded your eating or just read the dietary advice above, how could you eat differently in the fall and winter to keep your weight under control?

_____

_____

_____

Would you likely follow the same guidelines in spring and summer, or do you think you could relax your dietary controls and eat mainly what you want as you go along?

_____

_____

_____

Controlling your weight, exercising, and making wise use of supplements, while avoiding substances that can make SAD worse, is often an ongoing project. But with a series of small wins come big victories against the winter blues. Keep up the good work.

WHAT HAVE YOU LEARNED ABOUT DIET AND SAD?

Sometimes writing down what you gained (or where your expectations weren't met) helps gel your thoughts and stimulate new ideas. If you think it might help you plan for next year, jot down a few thoughts about any changes you want to make in diet and what you found easy and difficult about dietary changes you've already tried.

_____

_____

_____

Adding this information to your action plan in Chapter 6 can keep it useful as an up-to-date reference.

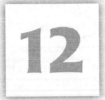

12

Transcending the Blues
Meditation and Relaxation

Tension can be a big factor in depression, affecting both mind and body. It's helpful to have some methods to ease it—and there is evidence that meditation can alleviate mood symptoms too.

Be Aware

WHAT DO YOU HOPE TO GET OUT OF MEDITATION AND/OR RELAXATION?

☐ No matter what I do, I feel edgy and tense and can barely handle the most minor hassles during the winter. I've got to find some new ways to manage stress so I can cope with my life at this time of year.

☐ I can't seem to stop beating myself up for how little I get done when I have active SAD symptoms. I'm hoping that meditating will help me let some of that go.

☐ I just thought I'd give meditation a try since I have friends who swear by it and say it's really easy to make into a habit.

☐ I feel like some joint or muscle is always stiff and sore in the winter and need to find a way to loosen up. I'm so tight that my balance and coordination seem off, and I feel like I'm bumping into things and falling a lot more easily. All I need to add to SAD is an injury!

Meditation and relaxation can benefit both the mind and the body. Meditation can help ease depression in a variety of ways, and different types of meditation can alleviate various symptoms. Relaxation can also be important to people with SAD, especially when stress and tension feel overwhelming. This chapter provides an overview of several types of meditation and then basic instructions for the method known as progressive relaxation.

MEDITATION

When practiced regularly, meditation changes the way both the brain and the body function. For people with SAD, meditation provides two main benefits:

1. *Meditation gives the nervous system a surge protector that helps prevent the surges triggered by recurrent stresses.* As you know, when you feel less stressed, your SAD symptoms improve.

2. *Meditation boosts creativity.* Leading a satisfying life with SAD often requires creative solutions. Ideas that eluded them at other times often come to people during transcendental meditation sessions, and mindfulness meditation can help clear away the mental and emotional static that blocks the flow of good ideas. In both cases, for example, you might stop agonizing over obligations that SAD symptoms prevent you from meeting and realize where help might be available.

↗ FAST FACTS

- Transcendental meditation increases the release of the soothing hormone prolactin, just as resting in the dark at night does, and lowers blood pressure and the risk of cardiovascular disease.

- Mindfulness meditation normalizes distressing emotions like sadness, preventing them from mushrooming into clinical depression.

- Loving-kindness compassion relieves the shame and guilt, and thereby lowers the resulting stress that depressed people often feel.

- Walking meditation combines light and exercise with meditation.

- Meditation eases anxiety as well as depression.

- Progressive relaxation is easy to learn and can be used anytime stress spirals out of control.

Debunking Myths about Meditation

- Meditation is not a religious practice (although it can be part of worship).

- Meditation does not require years of practice.

- Meditation does not require mysticism or spirituality—although it may become a mystical or spiritual experience for you. It can be performed by people of any religion or no religion at all.

- Meditation does not require you to go on lengthy retreats.

- Meditation is common in the West.

Although it involves the mind, the body, and the spirit, meditation is not that different from exercise in that you can decide how significant a role it should play in your life. Some people find meditating so transformative that their curiosity is piqued and they pursue knowledge and wisdom in the practice for the rest of their lives, in the same way that many fitness devotees and athletes build their skills and collect valuable self-knowledge and other insights as they push themselves to their physical and mental limits. Likewise, you can pursue meditation informally or via formal instruction (depending on the type of meditation), just as you can exercise on your own or at a gym with a trainer. For most people meditation is a helpful part of a full treatment regimen, but some people have gained so much benefit that meditation is a sufficient treatment for SAD by itself.

This chapter introduces you to transcendental meditation (TM), mindfulness, and loving-kindness. Each may be particularly useful for certain problems associated with SAD. Meditation of all kinds is largely free of side effects, requires little or no equipment, and in some cases no up-front expenses. The following questions and information might help you determine which form of meditation is most appealing to you.

Meditation and relaxation may be particularly helpful for summer SAD, which often causes agitation rather than depression.

Prepare

Which Type of Meditation Should You Try?

☐ Do you typically suffer anxiety and irritability along with the lows of depression during your SAD season?

→ **Transcendental meditation** is known to alleviate anxiety.

☐ Do you feel shame and constantly beat yourself up for being unable to surmount the effects of the seasons and "get on with life"?

→ **Loving-kindness meditation** focuses on developing the self-compassion to evaporate self-blame and guilt over things you cannot change (like having a biological vulnerability to the changes of season).

☐ Do you have a lot of trouble focusing on mental tasks?

→ **TM** is essentially an effortless method that may give you just the boost you need when the techniques involved in cognitive-behavioral therapy—a very effective intervention for depression—require more mental focus than you can manage. TM also improves attention and can help you achieve what you need to get done, which in turn will make you feel better about yourself if you're often down on yourself.

☐ Do you react to hassles with a hypersensitive fight-or-flight response?

→ **TM** can help here too, calming your autonomic nervous system in general.

☐ Do you feel like you're trudging along, shrouded in such dense fog during winter that you can't find joy or even contentment in anything, even when your depression symptoms are eased by other treatments?

→ **Mindfulness** trains you to become aware of your surroundings and your internal experience *in the moment* so that you can notice that pain waxes and wanes and there is often pleasure to be had even in the midst of sadness. With this awareness pleasant activities you pursue are more than token efforts and can help boost your mood when you're still not feeling as well as you'd like.

☐ Does SAD make you brood and ruminate, getting stuck in negative thoughts and self-blaming harangues?

→ **TM** seems to call a halt to the endless loop of negative thoughts.

→ **Mindfulness** teaches you to stay aware of how you feel physically and emotionally right now and watch negative thoughts pass by like clouds floating away in the sky.

☐ Is exhaustion a hallmark symptom of your SAD?

→ **TM** instills a state of restful alertness marked by the release of the hormone prolactin, which (as mentioned earlier in this book) is also released when we rest peacefully but awake in between long periods of sleep that occur when people stay in bed during the entire period of darkness during a winter night. This state can alleviate fatigue and restore energy lost to SAD.

☐ Do you find it impossible to ignore the bearing down of the cold darkness during a winter day?

→ **Mindfulness** opens your awareness to *all* that you are experiencing in the moment and to all the stimuli entering your consciousness. Instead of allowing your mind to keep poking you with the knowledge that it was so gloomy when you got up this morning, you'll be able to feel the sun peeking from behind the clouds, hear the music of the wind in the trees, marvel in the crystalline beauty of an icicle or a snowflake, and bask in the aromatic steam wafting from the pot of soup you have simmering on the stove.

☐ Does SAD make you feel outright antisocial?

→ **Loving-kindness meditation** helps you develop compassion toward yourself and then, naturally, to extend it to others. The isolation that often comes with SAD can make us feel vulnerable and in an inferior position, which can make us envy or resent those who don't have to deal with our challenges. It can also help us remind ourselves that any criticism directed at us for not "pulling our weight" in the winter is a result of ignorance rather than malice and cut off anger or more self-blame.

One or another of these three forms of meditation might also be best for practical reasons.

Instruction

TM requires formal instruction from a certified teacher, with this schedule of lessons:

1–2. Two roughly 1-hour public lectures to introduce what TM is. These are free of charge.

3. A 10-minute interview with a certified teacher.

4–7. One-on-one instruction from the teacher (1½–2 hours) one day, then three follow-up sessions (1–1½ hours each) on the next 3 days.

|▲| SCIENCE

Science Confirms the Benefits of TM

Transcendental meditation has proved so transformative for me and many others that I was moved to write a book about it. You'll find thorough coverage of the wealth of scientific research in its favor, as well as anecdotes that I hope will inspire you to consider this powerful tool in your SAD Solution arsenal, in *Transcendence* (see the Resources). TM has been shown in many clinical studies to lower stress, protect against heart disease, and strengthen psychological resilience, among its many other benefits.

* * *

Mindfulness meditation can be practiced both formally and informally. Self-help books are available to teach the practice of mindfulness, which you can then apply in scheduled sessions on your own (formal) as well as throughout the routine events of your day (informal). You can also attend formal group classes and retreats to learn or hone the practice of mindfulness. See the Resources at the back of the book for good books on the subject and sources of information on in-person instruction.

|▲| SCIENCE

Mindfulness-Based Cognitive Therapy for Depression

An intervention designed in 2002 that combines the practice of mindfulness meditation and CBT has been shown to cut risk of relapse of depression *by half* when mindfulness-based cognitive therapy (MBCT) was added to the treatment for depression patients were already receiving, particularly among those who had already had three or more episodes of depression. Although MBCT has not specifically been studied for use with SAD, the fact that for most people SAD has recurred for years might make this a very helpful form of therapy to seek out. MBCT has now shown the same significant benefits for relapse prevention in five randomized controlled studies. Because depression compromises the abilities necessary to do the work of CBT (which involves a lot of logging and writing homework), it's best to try to get the tools you can learn from MBCT in place during your best seasons and be prepared by wintertime. You can learn about MBCT in *The Mindful Way through Depression* and follow the 8-week program via self-help in *The Mindful Way Workbook,* both written by the originators of MBCT.

*   *   *

Loving-kindness meditation can also be practiced, at a simple level, via self-help, with the aid of books, websites, and audiovisual materials. Or you can seek out a private teacher, a group, or a meditation center that offers retreats and other training opportunities. See the Resources.

Costs

If you choose to learn mindfulness or loving-kindness via self-help, your costs obviously will be limited to the books or other resources you choose to use. You may also need a meditation bench and/or cushion, although you can even construct these inexpensively yourself. However, note that many experts believe you will get the maximum benefit from your practice if you have at least some formal training. The costs for group classes and retreats vary widely, depending on location and duration, among other factors.

TM requires specific instruction in seven steps, for which tuition is charged. You can find out what the tuition for the seven steps will be for your locale and your personal situation (employed or unemployed, student, veteran, age, etc.) by going to *www.tm.org* if you live in the United States or by searching the Internet for TM in your country. Note that the tuition can be paid over time and that the Transcendental Meditation Program is dedicated to trying to make tuition affordable through scholarships and other assistance if needed. Also, you can attend the first two presentations free of charge to find out whether you are interested in pursuing the program. You get a lot for your investment: once you have been trained, you have access to 20- to 30-minute follow-up sessions with a certified teacher wherever you live *for the rest of your life, without additional charge.*

Time

As noted above, you can practice mindfulness, and also loving-kindness, on a strictly informal basis, which means that you learn how to be mindful in the course of your daily routine. The goal in this case is to proceed as mindfully, with as much loving-kindness, as possible during your day. If you opt for formal mindfulness, for either type of mindfulness you should probably plan to spend 20–30 minutes twice a day. TM is done for 20 minutes twice a day, ideally early in the morning and late in the afternoon, before dinner. Mindfulness and loving-kindness can actually be integrated as one practice (see Christopher Germer's book *The Mindful Path to Self-Compassion*, listed in the Resources), and most experts recommend a minimum of 20 minutes per practice (once or twice a day) and up to 45 or 60 minutes if that seems workable and beneficial to you. But that is intended to give you the opportunity to ingrain the practice and its benefits; there is no harm in doing a shorter practice when that is all you can fit in.

What You Do during Meditation

Treat

Transcendental Meditation

> Paul was being treated effectively for seasonal bipolar disorder with medications, but managing symptoms wasn't enough to make him feel happy. TM stabilized his mood swings, calmed him, boosted his energy and enthusiasm, and helped him focus on tasks. After establishing a TM practice, he pronounced himself "truly happy 90% of the time."

For the 20 minutes of practice, you start by finding a peaceful, comfortable place where you can meditate uninterrupted—a quiet room where you can dim the lights and block out noise, with a comfortable place to sit. You get settled, close your eyes, and use your mantra—a specific sound or word—as previously instructed by a qualified TM teacher, transporting yourself to a mental state of peaceful alertness that typically brings (although this varies from person to person) profound relaxation, inner peace, and sometimes the intensely pleasurable shift in consciousness called *transcendence,* in which you seem to move beyond space and time into a state of pure bliss. Transcendence cannot be forced, and it may come and go. It may come with an enhanced sense of connection to others, which can make you feel supported without asking for support and decrease the isolation that people with SAD often feel because they are "different." During TM, practitioners experience measurable physical and neurological changes that exert beneficial effects on mood, blood pressure, emotional health, and much more. Many practitioners report that TM is, in truth, transformative. The peaceful state and physiological/neurological changes that occur during meditation also confer beneficial effects after the meditation session is over.

TM is an ineffable experience. The experience is different for different people and even varies within the same person from one session to the next. The brain is constantly changing, and the nature of the meditative experience will change along with it. Usually during meditation a person feels calm with slower breathing and a settling down within the body. At the same time the mind may experience a sense of deep rest or creative flashes or joy—or all of these. I encourage you, if you are intrigued, to attend one of the free lectures, which will at least provide you with an intellectual understanding of what you stand to gain and how. See *www.tm.com* or *www.davidlynchfoundation.com* to find a lecture and much more information. The David Lynch Foundation for Consciousness-Based Education and World Peace was formed in 2005 to fund the implementation of stress-reducing methods such as TM for at-risk populations around the world. You will also find many first-person descriptions of the experience and more details about what happens in the body and mind in my book *Transcendence*. The box on page 206 provides an excerpt of an interview with Bob Roth, a longtime TM instructor, that appeared in the book.

☀ *TM: A Pleasant Activity in and of Itself*

Learning mindfulness and developing self-compassion can, over time, help you build self-acceptance and attune yourself to the joys of life that may be hard to see through the shroud of SAD symptoms. Some people also find that they feel calm and peaceful after meditating. But mindfulness meditation can also bring up difficult feelings that you may have been trying to avoid. Mindfulness training does help you stay with these feelings until they pass naturally, which they will, and noting that they are transient can be very important to anyone who suffers from depression. Nevertheless, transcendental meditation does not typically involve such challenges, and in fact most people look forward to their meditation sessions as a pleasant activity.

TM sessions also add structure to your day. Because these sessions are pleasurable, practicing TM can become a kind of behavioral activation (a form of therapy that is designed to overcome inertia by adding positively reinforcing activities to your life; more on this in Chapter 13). Having things to do—and doing them—increases the feeling of competence and thus can boost self-esteem, something those with SAD often find themselves lacking.

How Does TM Work?

From an interview with Bob Roth, who has been teaching TM around the world for more than 40 years:

The transcendental meditation technique makes use of the mind's natural tendency to be drawn—or attracted—toward fields of greater charm or satisfaction. For example, you are sitting in a room listening to music, but the music is not very good, so you're easily distracted. Then some beautiful music comes wafting in from another room. What happens? Your attention spontaneously shifts from the not-so-pleasing music to the really good music. And it's the same with books. If you're deep in a really great book, you could be anywhere—in a crowded airport, waiting for hours—and your attention will stay right there on the page. We infer that deep within the mind, at the very source of thought, is a reservoir of energy, intelligence, and happiness. You would logically expect that this field would be an incredibly satisfying place to "be," and it is. After all, it is your own inner Self.

When you learn TM, you learn a technique that reliably turns the attention of your mind within. It's like leaning over to dive into a pool—once you're in the right position, the movement just naturally happens. With no effort at all, your attention moves to increasingly subtle, quiet, creative, and energetic levels of the mind. How do you know this is happening? Because the mind and body are connected, and you can feel it. As the mind is settling down during TM practice, the body must likewise be gaining a state of deep rest, and the functioning of the brain must change as well. And that is exactly what the research shows. During the TM technique the body is deeply rested and the mind is settled yet wide awake. You're in a unique, yet completely natural state of restful alertness. It's far different from simply resting with your eyes closed.

|▲| SCIENCE

Can TM Make You More Effective?

Apparently it can—by increasing *coherence* across the brain between alpha and beta brain wave activity, even in TM newcomers. Coherence is associated with higher intelligence and competence (highly successful business managers in Norway had greater coherence than coworkers who were skilled and knowledgeable but had no management responsibilities, and elite athletes had greater coherence than those who didn't compete as well, in two studies). The increased coherence during TM occurs in the prefrontal lobes of the brain, the command center for both decision making and emotional regulation. In other words, TM improves mood *and* mental capacities.

The longer you continue your TM practice, the more likely that you'll experience increased coherence *after* meditation, meaning your session in the morning might make you more focused and effective throughout the day.

⚠ *End TM Sessions Gradually!*

Although side effects are virtually nonexistent, those who have had TM sessions interrupted or who have tried to emerge from meditating abruptly sometimes experience headaches. So it's important to schedule your sessions at a time and in a place where you are least likely to be interrupted. It's also best not to meditate right before you go to bed, which can produce one of the few other side effects: disturbing dreams.

Mindfulness and Loving-Kindness Meditation

Helen finds that breathing, insight, and loving-kindess meditations help her achieve equanimity through an understanding that all things, including emotional distress, pass. Using light therapy first thing in the morning helped her focus on meditation, which she did directly afterward.

Danilo had found light therapy and adding exercise to his day very helpful with his SAD symptoms, but he often skipped one or the other or both, berating himself for taking time away from all the things he had to get done and then feeling even worse about himself when his symptoms intensified and his productivity plummeted. Through loving-kindness meditation he recognized the value of self-compassion and began to develop a deeper, more forgiving acceptance of SAD's limitations on him.

As noted above, you can meditate using these practices both formally and informally. During a formal meditation session you typically sit or kneel comfortably (heels resting on the backs of your legs) on a meditation cushion and prepare yourself by doing a deep breathing exercise. You might follow with a type of exercise called a *body scan* to tune your consciousness in to the physical feelings you are experiencing—tightness here, ache there, tickle here, itch there. During the body scan you learn to gently approach these feelings and ask yourself about their source: Is there an emotion that resides there that you've been unaware of? While continuing with intentional breathing, you let yourself become fully aware of all the sensations and thoughts and other aspects of your internal experience that come to you, all the while accepting them, inviting your mind to explore them gently, but also letting them move on according to their natural expiration. A major goal of mindfulness is to train us to accept whatever is occurring—whether painful or pleasurable—while it is occurring, because it is resistance that, ironically, perpetuates emotional pain. In the words of psychologist Christopher Germer and many others, self-blame, asking ourselves why we can't just feel better, numbing, pretending that we are not experiencing what we are experiencing—all of these very human reactions by which we try to push away discomfort—compound pain and turn it into suffering. With mindful awareness, we can learn from our pain ("What can I do differently that will minimize avoidable pain in the future?") without getting trapped in it.

Mindlessness, the opposite of mindfulness, is rampant. How many times have you . . .

- ☐ **Driven to your local supermarket, only to arrive in the parking lot and realize you couldn't remember getting there?**

- ☐ **Bolted down a fast-food lunch without tasting a thing?**

- ☐ **Read a page of a novel you thought you were enjoying, only to find that you didn't absorb a word because you were busy writing tomorrow's to-do list in your head or rehashing yesterday's argument?**

- ☐ **Gone to a different room in your house or office to get something and had no idea why you were there when you arrived?**

- ☐ **Felt miserable while doing an easy chore because you were grumbling throughout about having to do it?**

To get a very simple look at the difference between mindlessness and the experience of mindfulness, try the exercises on pages 210 and 211 if you like. The raisin exercise will give you an idea of how little attention we pay even to an experience that is entirely sensory, like eating. Try the raisin exercise once and then, if you found it illuminating, do it again with another raisin to see how much more you notice the second time around.

Christopher Germer suggests that you try the following mindful walking exercise first at home, very slowly, and then again outdoors on one of your normal routes. Walking mindfully in a beautiful natural environment will allow you to appreciate the full panoply of sensory delights that you might ordinarily ignore.

Marjorie engages in mindful walking in London's beautiful Kew Gardens. Although being outdoors in gorgeous surroundings (sometimes in sunshine) may be somewhat helpful to her SAD symptoms, without mindfulness she found such walks encouraged her to dwell on negative thoughts. Mindfulness helps her relax and return home with less stress.

What Have You Learned from Experimenting with Mindfulness?

If you have time right after doing the raisin or walking exercise (or both), jot down some thoughts about what you discovered. What did your senses tell you that you never noticed before? How did you feel during and after the exercises?

_____

_____

_____

_____

Did what you learned make you want to delve more deeply into mindfulness? If so, you might want to read more:

- *The Mindful Way through Depression* and *The Mindful Path to Self-Compassion* are both great sources of information, inspiration, and instruction. Both contain lists of meditation centers and other resources where you can seek in-person training.

- *The Mindful Way Workbook: An 8-Week Program to Free Yourself from Depression and Emotional Distress,* by John Teasdale, Zindel Segal, and Mark Williams. This workbook is based on the 8-week MBCT program that has proven so

The Raisin Exercise: A First Taste of Mindfulness

1. Holding

First, take a raisin and hold it in the palm of your hand or between your finger and thumb.

Focusing on it, imagine that you've just dropped in from Mars and have never seen an object like this before in your life.

2. Seeing

Take time to really see it; gaze at it with care and full attention.

Let your eyes explore every part of it, examining the highlights where the light shines, the darker hollows, the folds and ridges, any asymmetries or unique features.

3. Touching

Turn it over between your fingers, exploring its texture, maybe with your eyes closed if that enhances your sense of touch.

4. Smelling

Holding it beneath your nose, with each inhalation drink in any aroma that may arise, noticing as you do this anything interesting that may be happening in your mouth or stomach.

5. Placing

Now slowly bring the raisin up to your lips, noticing how your hand and arm know exactly how and where to position it. Gently place the object in the mouth, without chewing, noticing how it gets into the mouth in the first place. Spend a few moments exploring the sensations of having it in your mouth, exploring it with your tongue.

6. Tasting

When you are ready, prepare to chew it, noticing how and where it needs to be for chewing. Then, very consciously, take one or two bites into it and notice what happens in the aftermath, experiencing any waves of taste that emanate from it as you continue chewing. Without swallowing yet, notice the bare sensations of taste and texture in the mouth and how these may change over time, moment by moment, as well as any changes in the object itself.

7. Swallowing

When you feel ready to swallow, see if you can first detect the intention to swallow as it comes up, so that even this is experienced consciously before you actually swallow the raisin.

8. Following

Finally, see if you can feel what is left of it moving down into your stomach, and sense how the body as a whole is feeling after completing this exercise in mindful eating.

effective in preventing recurrences of major depression and can be used either on your own or with a group led by a trained expert (see Resources).

- *The Mindfulness Solution: Everyday Practices for Everyday Problems,* by Ronald D. Siegel, contains an excellent chapter on using mindfulness to help with depression, including becoming more tuned in to all of your emotions—not just those associated with SAD symptoms. Becoming aware of your positive reactions to specific events, activities, and environments can give you valuable information about the pleasant activities to pursue and the mood-lifting measures you can take to ease your seasonal problems.

Mindful Walking

Plan to walk for 10 minutes or longer. Find a quiet place in your home where you can walk back and forth at least 10–20 feet at a time, or in a circle. Decide to use the time to cultivate moment-to-moment, kindly awareness.

- Stand still for a moment and anchor your attention in your body. Be aware of yourself in the standing posture. Feel your body.

- Start to walk slowly and deliberately. Notice how it feels to lift one foot, step forward, and place it down as the other foot begins to lift off the floor. Do the same with the other foot. Feel the sensations of lifting, stepping, and placing, over and over again. Feel free to use the words *lift, step, place* to focus your attention on the task.

- When your mind wanders, gently return to the physical sensations of walking. If you feel any urgency to move faster, simply note that and return to the sensations of walking.

- Do this with kindness and gratitude. Your relatively small feet are supporting your entire body; your hips are supporting your whole torso. Experience the marvel of walking.

- Move slowly and fluidly through space, being aware that you're walking. Some people find it easiest to keep their attention below the knees, or exclusively on the soles of the feet.

- When you reach the end of your walking space, pause a moment, take a conscious breath, remain anchored in your body, and reverse direction.

- At the end of the meditation period, invite yourself to be mindful of body sensations throughout the day. Notice the sensations of walking as you go on to your next activity.

The self-compassion developed through loving-kindness meditation is also a boon to SAD sufferers. Even if you've made progress in accepting your condition and the fact that it prevents you from doing everything you might like to do during your low time of year, the ugly finger of self-blame probably ends up pointed at you now and then. If so, or even just to get through the feeling of sorrow that this disorder has imposed a limitation on you, you might try using a self-compassion mantra. You can use the following phrase in a formal 20-minute meditation practice or anytime during the course of your day when you feel guilt or shame or sorrow or anger at having SAD, or if anything else is making you feel negative emotions:

May I be safe.

May I be happy.

May I be healthy.

May I live my life with ease.

Feel free to vary the words to make them more personally meaningful, such as adding or substituting "May I be free from suffering" for one of the lines. An audio download of the full exercise is available at *www.mindfulselfcompassion.org*. But you might experiment with simply repeating this mantra over and over at any time you feel bad about having SAD and see if it makes you feel better about yourself.

⚠ *Don't Expect Mindful Self-Compassion to Instill Good Feelings!*

The goal of self-compassion is to instill good *will* toward yourself—to muffle the voice of self-blame that nags so many people with SAD. Using loving-kindness meditation to try to feel happy and carefree will lead nowhere—it may even make you feel worse when those feelings don't materialize. You may, however, gain a sense of peace and self-acceptance from this form of meditation.

RELAXATION

Not all stress can be eliminated through the methods described in Chapter 9, such as time management. There are some stressors we can't avoid, and, unfortunately, depressive conditions, like SAD, are often accompanied by anxiety. Therefore having some tools to induce relaxation is important. Relaxation often results from meditation, but at least for mindfulness and loving-kindness, it's not the goal. Other ways to achieve relaxation:

- The deep breathing that you may learn in meditation training

- Biofeedback (ask your therapist if you're interested)

- Various forms of yoga

- Visualization

- Self-hypnosis

One method that many people find useful to learn is *progressive muscle relaxation*. This is a good technique to try when you find yourself ruminating and tied up in knots at any moment. You'll need to sit down or lie down in a quiet place, but other than that the technique can be used just about anywhere.

Progressive Muscle Relaxation

Treat

This technique has been widely used since the 1930s, when it was developed by an American physician named Edmund Jacobson. Like meditation, its positive effects increase with practice. Progressive relaxation ideally should take 20 to 30 minutes, but shortened versions can also be useful.

Start by finding a quiet place where you can lie down or sit comfortably. Remove your glasses or contacts, loosen any tight clothing, and rest your hands on your lap or at your side (or on the arms of your chair).

What you are going to do is tense and then relax each group of muscles, starting with your feet and moving upward to your head or vice versa. Choose whichever sequence seems more natural to you. Because we so often carry our tension in the head and neck, many people find it more useful to start there and work down the body.

You can vary the time for holding the tension and then relaxation. Some instructions call for tensing the muscles for 15 seconds and then relaxing for 30; others for tensing for 5 seconds and relaxing for 20; and still others for tensing while you count to 5 and then relaxing while you count to 10. You can choose the time intervals that work best for you, but while you are learning the technique, the longer times will allow you more time to notice the feelings of tensing and relaxing. This mental aspect of the technique is critical—the feeling of a relaxed muscle becomes associated with relaxation in general, so that you can elicit mental relaxation when necessary to counteract rising anxiety by relaxing certain muscle groups.

1. Take a few slow, deep breaths, concentrating only on inhaling and exhaling. Try to breathe from the diaphragm (see page 215).

2. Head: You can do this either with your whole face or with your forehead and then your jaw. Tense all the muscles in your face (squeeze your eyes closed, clamp your jaw shut, press your lips together in a frown) or in your forehead as you slowly inhale to a count of anywhere from 5 to 15. Focus on tensing only those muscles. While slowly exhaling, release the tension, relaxing the same muscles gradually over 10–30 seconds. Pause for a few seconds once the muscles are completely relaxed. (If you started with the forehead, now do the same with your jaw.)

3. Neck and shoulders: Now tense and relax your neck and shoulders in the same way, for the same time intervals. Repeat with the remaining muscle groups . . .

4. Chest.

5. Stomach/abdomen.

6. Right arm and hand: first the whole arm, then making a fist with the right forearm and hand, then just the hand.

7. Left arm and hand: first the whole arm, then making a fist with the left forearm and hand, and then just the hand.

8. Buttocks.

9. Right leg and foot: first the whole leg, then the lower leg and foot, then just the foot.

10. Left leg and foot: first the whole leg, then the lower leg and foot, then just the foot.

Variations

• *Shorter version:* Once you've learned the technique, or when you're short of time, you can tense and relax just the four main muscle groups: (1) face/head; (2) neck, shoulders, arms, and hands; (3) abdomen and chest; (4) buttocks, legs, and feet.

• *With audio:* You can find many scripts for progressive muscle relaxation online that you could record yourself (or ask someone whose voice you find soothing to record the script for you) and then listen to during practice. Audio downloads are also available online.

- *With visualization:* Some people find that visualizing a pleasant, soothing scene promotes relaxation during the exercise. You might imagine you're floating on a cloud, noticing the beautiful scenery as you drift over it, whether that's a bubbling stream, a field filled with wildflowers and gently chirping birds, or a sun-drenched beach. For those with SAD, it can be particularly helpful to visualize the sun and imagine that you have control over the sunlight, directing it over each muscle group as you relax it. Visualization is most useful when you train all your senses on what you are imagining.

Diaphragmatic Breathing

Treat

Deep breathing from the abdomen rather than the chest promotes relaxation. Quick, shallow breathing is usually associated with anxiety and tension. To recognize the difference, try lying on your back with your hands resting gently on your abdomen. Slowly inhale, trying to push the air into your abdomen instead of your chest. If you're breathing from the diaphragm, your hands will rise as your lower abdomen expands with air. If you're breathing from the chest, your chest will rise and your rib cage will expand. (You can also put one hand on your chest and one on your abdomen. The hand on your chest should not move if you are breathing from the diaphragm.)

Just Breathe!

Deep, slow breathing is so important to relaxation. It's critical during exercise, delivering more oxygen to your muscles and expelling carbon dioxide as you work out than shallow breathing does. For most of us, our fallback breathing method is shallow. Change that and you may not only become calm more often but also feel more energetic (from the extra oxygen).

First, learn to recognize the physical pang that typically accompanies anxiety. Many people feel it in the pit of their stomach or in their chest. It feels like fear, with a big physical twinge. Often you'll notice that you instinctively take a quick breath at the same time; that's your body trying to get a little extra oxygen to prepare for fight or flight. If you can train yourself to recognize this event and immediately follow it with the silent command to yourself, "Breathe," the shift to deep breathing will eventually become automatic, and anxiety will have a harder time getting a hold on you. Mindfulness meditation is a good medium in which to recognize pangs of anxiety.

Fortunately, just 1–3 minutes of breathing will calm you down and can be done anywhere without anyone else knowing you're doing anything differently at all. Try it at these times just to get used to shifting into it whenever you can:

- **While walking: It can really help you take in your surroundings and enhance the relaxation response.**

- **During meetings: Feeling antsy? Irritable? Bored and tired? Shift to deep breathing and get back your calm and your energy.**

- **While trying to fall asleep: Especially if your sleep is often interrupted by ruminative thoughts, focusing on diaphragmatic breathing is a good way to relax, get out of your head, and get back to sleep.**

- **When nervous: Even if you don't spot the physiological signs of anxiety, in situations that might make you feel a little nervous, it's a good idea to prepare by doing some deep breathing in advance.**

What Have You Learned about Meditation and Relaxation?

Sometimes writing down what you gained (or where your expectations weren't met) helps gel your thoughts and stimulate new ideas. If you think it might help you plan for next year, jot down a few thoughts about what type of meditation or progressive relaxation you'd like to pursue or how you benefited from anything after you've tried it.

_____

_____

_____

Adding this information to your action plan in Chapter 6 can keep it useful as an up-to-date reference.

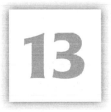

Finding Your Happiness

Pleasant Activities

Easing SAD symptoms isn't enough to replace the contentment and joy lost to depression. We need to make an intentional effort to add pleasant activities to our daily lives.

This chapter and the next one present a potent selection of remedies based on cognitive-behavioral therapy, shown to be one of the most effective treatments for depression to date. As with Chapters 10 and 11, the strategies in Chapters 13 and 14 support each other and therefore work best in concert, but you can cherry-pick the ones that will give you those all-important small wins and then add tools as desired. Cognitive-behavioral therapy (CBT) is based on the premise that our thoughts drive our behavior and our behaviors in turn affect our thoughts—and our emotions go along for the ride. In depression, negative thoughts and beliefs keep low mood entrenched and prevent us from engaging in behaviors that would alleviate the blues. Why not get started right now in learning how you might adjust your thinking and choose behaviors that will make your life a lot less SAD?

Be Aware

WHAT DO YOU HOPE TO GET FROM CHANGING NEGATIVE THOUGHTS AND PURSUING PLEASANT ACTIVITIES?

☐ I want to figure out why my life still feels unfulfilling even though light and other treatments have resolved most of my SAD symptoms.

☐ I want to start looking forward to and planning for the future—instead of dreading winter every year—for the first time in my life.

☐ I want to be happy.

☐ SAD is still bothering me despite some improvements, and before I consider medication, I want to see whether something else is standing in my way of feeling a lot better.

☐ Light therapy hasn't done much for me, and I don't want to take medications. I'm willing to do some work to resolve my SAD symptoms.

☐ Light therapy helps me a lot during the fall and winter, but then, the next year, here comes SAD again. Is there any way to break this vicious cycle?

☐ I just want to have some fun, like everyone else.

↗ FAST FACTS

- Negative thinking tends to create self-fulfilling prophecies of doom ("I'm going to feel miserable all winter," because it assumes there's nothing you can do, leads you to do nothing, and you keep on feeling miserable).

- CBT provides entry points into thoughts, emotions, and behavior where positive change in one area can create positive change in the others.

- A few well-controlled studies have shown CBT to be effective specifically in SAD; hundreds have shown CBT to help significantly with depression generally.

- You can build concrete skills to eliminate negative thoughts and improve mood.

- Parts of the brain involved in negative thinking seem to calm down after CBT, whereas parts involved in positive emotions become more active.

- Depression discourages us from pursuing pleasant activities, but actively participating in them actually alleviates depression.

⚗ SCIENCE

CBT for SAD

Thanks to associate professor of psychology Kelly Rohan and colleagues, CBT has been compared in research to light therapy alone and to a combination of CBT and light therapy in treating SAD. All three treatments proved effective, but those who had received CBT had lower relapse rates the following winter than those who had not. My guess is that CBT outperformed light therapy in preventing relapse the next winter because it encouraged pleasant activities but also improved consciousness and thoughtfulness about the condition itself—both essential to optimal treatment. Again, synergy = energy.

Let's start with the fun.

ADDING PLEASANT ACTIVITIES

In CBT, we look at how thoughts, behavior, and emotions are interconnected. Think about your experience with SAD: The way you go about your day obviously has an effect on your SAD symptoms. Take sleeping late as an example. You sleep in, which makes you miss out on your pre-breakfast walk outside or fitting in light therapy at the time of day when it's most effective. This makes your SAD symptoms worse, and when your depression worsens, you're more likely to sleep in again.

⚠️ *Don't Let Anything Keep You in Bed Late!*

Yielding to the depression-driven temptation to sleep in creates a vicious cycle of worsening SAD symptoms: You miss out on the therapeutic early-morning sunlight, and maybe also on your scheduled light therapy, which drives your mood downward, which feeds the urge to sleep more. . . . So do whatever it takes to get up on time: set three alarm clocks, ask a family member to wake you, have a friend give you a wake-up call, use a dawn simulator (see Chapter 7).

As a second example, let's say you stay at your desk all day, struggling to pay this month's bills, despite the fact that you're tired and having trouble concentrating and keep losing your focus on the task at hand. Not finishing the job makes you feel guilty and disgusted with yourself, so you refuse to meet your friend for afternoon coffee as planned and then spend the evening feeling miserable and alone. The next day you wake up already feeling like a "loser," so depressed you still can't finish the bill paying.

Behavior → Thoughts → Emotions

It's important to know what behaviors you engage in that might actually make your symptoms worse. Think over days that just seemed to go downhill during the season when your symptoms are active. Can you identify anything you did (or didn't do, like refusing to go out for coffee) that made you feel worse? List some ideas here:

_____

_____

_____

_____

_____

What you wrote down could include anything from sleeping late or bowing out of social plans to skipping light therapy or medication, spending too much time in a dark indoor space, forgoing exercise, or trying to fit the same tasks and chores into a winter day as you can fit into a summer day.

Now let's focus on that second scenario, the one in which a person with SAD punishes himself for not getting an important chore done by denying himself a pleasant activity. People with SAD deny themselves fun for so many different reasons. Which ones have you adopted?

☐ I haven't gotten enough done today, so I shouldn't waste time on frivolity.

☐ I'm too tired.

☐ I just can't seem to enjoy the things I used to.

☐ I'm too crabby to be around other people.

☐ *Nothing* sounds like fun to me.

☐ Doing anything beyond my obligations exhausts me even more.

☐ Winter is never going to be fun for me. I just have to have my fun in the summer.

All these reasons are founded in assumptions that may not be true and therefore should not be relied on as factual, especially because they actually keep you from a legitimate form of treatment for SAD: *pleasant activities*. Let's say the woman who slept late loves her morning walks not just for the symptom-reducing effects of the early-morning sun and the exercise but because the outdoors makes her feel calm and she always runs into dog walkers, and she loves dogs. When she comes back from her walk, she feels a surge of happiness and energy that keeps her going for much of the day. Now picture the man who denies himself a coffee date. If he had kept that date, knowing that the social connection would break up an unpleasant task and make him feel less isolated, he would have felt less depressed that day and the next morning. If they had paid attention to this sequence, both people might have developed different beliefs: "Dragging myself out of bed will pay off." "I deserve to go out and have a little fun, and it will make me more productive if I do." So the reverse phenomenon is also true:

Emotions → Thoughts → Behavior

In fact, this sequence is really a circle, and it operates both clockwise and counterclockwise. Pleasant activities are self-reinforcing. When you pursue them often enough, your brain has the chance to learn that they make you feel better, and as a result you're more likely to pursue them again—and feel even better as their beneficial effects accumulate.

As with exercise and other active pursuits, you may not believe this until you experience it for yourself. So I'm going to ask you to make a promise to yourself that you won't regret:

I vow to spend at least 10 minutes every day in a pleasant activity.

Ten minutes is hardly any time at all, and yet you're probably aware of how a whole day can slip away in the fog of SAD or in the exhausting, futile effort to meet obligations you don't have the energy for.

Erase the Objections

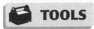

Perhaps my attempt to extract that promise from you is already raising the din of objections like those you checked off above. If so, you can use a time-honored CBT tool called *self-talk*.

TOOLS

Tools You Can Use: Positive Self-Talk

Feel like you don't have the luxury of spending time on fun? Tell yourself:

"I deserve a little fun, just like everyone else."

Too tired? Tell yourself:

> *"I can push through it, and I'll end up feeling better."*

Lost the ability to feel pleasure? Tell yourself:

> *"Do it anyway. Pleasure will come back to me over time."*

Too grumpy to be around other people? Tell yourself:

> *"My friends/family always make me laugh. I'll be able to muffle the crabbiness enough to be civil."*

Can't figure out what could possibly feel pleasant to do? Tell yourself:

> *"I'll try something, and if it doesn't work out, I'll note that and try something else."*

Anything you add to your day ends up just making you more tired? Tell yourself:

> *"A little bit of fun is always energizing emotionally even if tiring physically."*

Giving up on winter? Tell yourself:

> *"Winter may never feel like summer to me, but it sure can get better than this."*

Self-talk takes practice, as do all CBT techniques. To be sure you use it, you might consider writing down some simple messages like those above, or even a phrase as fundamental as "I can do it" or "Get started and I'll be able to keep going" to carry around with you—use an index card you can put in your pocket or enter your self-talk into your smartphone. Whenever you hear one of the anti-pleasure excuses arise in your mind, read your self-talk message to yourself.

While we're on the subject of behavior, there are ways besides self-talk to erase the objections above—change something else you do:

- One key behavior is to manage your time using the stress management tips in Chapter 9. That is, use other resources (like the help of family and friends) to cut down on your daily obligations in winter so that you have a window available for pleasant activities.

- If fatigue is a huge problem for you, see what you can do to bump up your energy (understanding that SAD is going to make you tired but there are things that might counteract some fatigue): Get more light, or earlier light? Take vitamins? Cut out alcohol? Start exercising if you haven't done so already? (There is more on these possibilities in Chapter 10.) Stop staying up late watching movies? As mentioned earlier in the book, this doesn't mean giving up a pleasant activity but simply scheduling it when it won't do more harm than good.

Treat

Pick Your Pleasure Carefully

Because depression can rob you of motivation, self-awareness, energy, and the ability to feel enjoyment, it's helpful to take a systematic approach to reintroducing pleasant activities into your life.

1. *Choose some activities that you've enjoyed in the past or think you would enjoy now.* You can find lists of hundreds of possible activities online (search for "pleasant events schedule" or "pleasant activities lists" or the like), but to make this initial step a little easier, I've compiled a list of 80 activities in the form on page 224. Pick a moment when you're feeling relatively peaceful and alert and quickly run down the list, checking off any activity that sounds appealing. Don't give this too much thought now; you can narrow down the list later.

2. *Circle the activities that would be easy to do right away (those that take little preparation and that can be done in as little as 10 minutes).*

3. *Now decide on one activity you could do—and would like to do—each day this week for at least 10 minutes.* You can use the Pleasant Activities Log on page 225 if you like. Otherwise, just refer back to your circled activities each morning and pick one to pursue that day. If you're using the log, check off the activity once you've done it, give it an enjoyment rating on a scale of 1–10, and if you think it will help you pursue the most pleasant, stress-free activities for you, add comments: When and where did you do the activity? For how long? What you would do the same or differently next time (e.g., repeat that activity or choose something else)? Did the activity change your mood? (You can also enter that last comment on your Daily Mood Log if you're using it regularly.)

SCIENCE

Happiness and sadness are not two sides of the same coin. Many people believe that if only they eased their depression they would be deliriously happy. Not

Pleasant Activities Checklist

- ☐ Taking a hot shower or bath
- ☐ Watching TV
- ☐ Gardening
- ☐ Reading a book
- ☐ Taking a walk
- ☐ Flirting
- ☐ Going somewhere to watch a sport
- ☐ Playing a card game
- ☐ Going to a concert
- ☐ Cooking dinner
- ☐ Taking a scenic drive
- ☐ Painting, sculpting, or other art
- ☐ Dressing up
- ☐ Pleasing my partner
- ☐ Attending a religious service
- ☐ Talking to a friend on the phone
- ☐ Surprising my children
- ☐ Listening to music
- ☐ Having a party
- ☐ Taking care of my parents
- ☐ Eating a fancy chocolate
- ☐ Sitting on the beach
- ☐ Having a picnic
- ☐ Napping
- ☐ Going to a beauty salon
- ☐ Shopping
- ☐ Petting my dog

- ☐ Riding my bike
- ☐ Going to a flea market
- ☐ Cleaning the house
- ☐ Rearranging furniture
- ☐ Cuddling with the cat
- ☐ Playing the piano (or other musical instrument)
- ☐ Problem solving
- ☐ Daydreaming
- ☐ Baking cookies (or a cake or pie)
- ☐ Meeting someone for coffee
- ☐ Playing an interactive game on the computer
- ☐ Looking up exotic locations online
- ☐ Dancing
- ☐ Filing
- ☐ Writing letters or e-mails
- ☐ Laughing with a friend
- ☐ Watching a movie
- ☐ Ironing
- ☐ Giving advice
- ☐ Volunteering
- ☐ Tutoring
- ☐ Coaching a sport
- ☐ Playing a team sport
- ☐ Planning a vacation
- ☐ Singing in a choir
- ☐ Collecting
- ☐ Having a massage

- ☐ Discussing philosophy, history, or another subject
- ☐ Raking leaves
- ☐ Playing cards
- ☐ Having sex
- ☐ Performing in front of others
- ☐ Jogging
- ☐ Doing carpentry or building
- ☐ Giving gifts
- ☐ Doing puzzles (jigsaw, sudoku, other)
- ☐ Creative writing
- ☐ Taking a class
- ☐ Having a special glass of wine
- ☐ Swimming
- ☐ Taking photos
- ☐ Using social networking sites
- ☐ Going to a museum
- ☐ Having tea
- ☐ Planning meals
- ☐ Taking care of personal finances
- ☐ Stargazing
- ☐ Eating in a restaurant
- ☐ Playing solitaire
- ☐ Playing golf
- ☐ Going bowling
- ☐ Praying
- ☐ Reading or watching the news

Pleasant Activities Log

Day	Activity	Done (✓)	How enjoyable? (1–10)	Comments
Sunday				
Monday				
Tuesday				
Wednesday				
Thursday				
Friday				
Saturday				

true, according to the latest psychological studies. Efforts to ease depression do just that—ease depression. If you want to be happy, add pleasant activities.

Tips for Scheduling Pleasant Activities—*and Following Through*

- **Start small** if you can't seem to feel pleasure in anything. Pick something you enjoyed in the past and do it for just a few minutes at first—like taking 5 minutes to flip through your favorite magazine. With repetition, enjoyment will build.

- **Don't exclude things that aren't necessarily "fun and games" but that give you**

a sense of accomplishment. Even a small win like neatening your desk or making a bed can feel enjoyable and should be pursued.

- **Break up longer activities into pieces.** Do you love shopping but feel guilty taking an afternoon? Stop at one of your favorite shops on the way home from an errand and allow yourself 10 minutes of browsing. Do you enjoy housecleaning but feel exhausted just thinking about scrubbing down every room? Pick one room to dust and declutter—whatever you can do in 10 minutes.

- **Make your pleasant activities a high priority**—as high, in fact, as your work, chores, and errands. Think of pleasant activities as "appointments with fun" and take them as seriously as you would an appointment with your doctor or the deadline for a report. This should be easy to do if you start with committing to only 10 minutes a day.

- **Fine-tune your plan and add more pleasant activities** as the pleasure you take in these activities reinforces these new behaviors. The ultimate goal is to reach a good balance between the necessary and the enjoyable.

Troubleshooting: What If You Didn't Enjoy the Activities You Chose?

☐ **Did you choose the wrong time of day for this activity? (If, for example, you sat down for a cup of tea and a scone in the morning and took a walk in the late afternoon and found both activities draining, try reversing their time slots.)**

☐ **Did you choose the wrong activity? (Maybe brisk hikes just won't work for you in the winter even though you enjoy them tremendously in summer. Perhaps you decided to watch a movie that your cousin swore was hilarious and you just ended up bored because it really wasn't the type of movie you'd ever choose on your own.)**

WHAT HAVE YOU LEARNED ABOUT INCORPORATING PLEASANT ACTIVITIES INTO YOUR DAILY LIFE?

Sometimes writing down what you gained (or where your expectations weren't met) helps gel your thoughts and stimulate new ideas. If you think it might help you plan for next year, jot down some thoughts about what you've learned about yourself by starting to explore CBT and how you can plan to keep pleasant activities in your life during fall and winter.

_____

_____

_____

Adding this information to your action plan in Chapter 6 can keep it useful as an up-to-date reference.

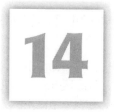

Using Your Head
Helpful Thoughts

(Re)learning your ABCs—the connection between the Antecedent (an event), the Belief triggered, and the Consequence (an emotion)—is among the most important things you can do to beat SAD. Cognitive-behavioral therapy (CBT), even in self-help form, may be enough to help you cope with and, in effect, treat your SAD symptoms without light therapy or medication. Even if you simply become aware of the connection between events, thoughts, and emotions, you can gain a lot of insights that will help you cope with SAD.

With this strong endorsement in mind, it makes sense to consider incorporating CBT into your SAD Solution APP. If you decided to add pleasant activities to your life using some of the ideas in Chapter 13, you may not need any convincing to consider the tools in this chapter. Numerous reliable studies have shown CBT to be effective for depression and also specifically for SAD. (See Chapter 12 for more on MBCT, a sort of hybrid of CBT and mindfulness meditation, which is also highly effective with depression.) And you don't need to sign on for a full course of CBT to benefit. You can pick and choose CBT strategies from this chapter the same way you can cherry-pick the tools in the whole workbook. And keep in mind that, even though some writing is involved in CBT, so is a lot of enjoyment that you have undoubtedly been missing out on.

HELPFUL THOUGHTS

What are helpful thoughts? They're thoughts that are not negative, automatic, distorted, or based on negative core beliefs. You'll notice I didn't say that helpful thoughts are *positive* thoughts. They might be positive, but they don't need to be—and they certainly don't need to sound like they came out of the mouth of Pollyanna. Helpful thoughts are rational and well considered instead of knee-jerk responses, based on realistic expectations and beliefs.

Automatic negative thoughts (aptly known as ANTs, considering the pests they can be) are the engine that drives much of depression, which is why they are the number-one target of CBT and may be why CBT alone can make deep inroads into SAD symptoms: Get rid of ANTs and depression's hold on you is loosened. (This is also one way that meditation helps: it tends to reduce automatic negative thoughts and promote helpful thoughts.)

One way that ANTs can worsen or at least perpetuate depression can be seen in the thoughts that you may have when you consider pursuing pleasant activities. Take a look at an example:

Antecedent: Your wife suggests that you call your brother and see whether he wants to go to the gym with you.

Automatic negative thought: "I can't do that; I'm way too tired and no fun to be around."

Consequence: The emotional consequence is that you feel ashamed of your limitations. Or maybe you feel angry that your wife doesn't understand how hard it is for you to go out and do something active. Either way, the behavioral consequence of that emotion is that you snap back that you're not up to it. Therefore you miss out on energizing exercise, a spirit-lifting change of scene, doing something you enjoy (working out), and socializing with someone who's fun to spend time with. Instead of feeling better that afternoon, you feel even worse.

ANTs can also rear their ugly little heads in parts of your life that aren't directly related to SAD. In a classic example of how our automatic negative thoughts can affect our mood and emotions, a woman is walking down the sidewalk and spots a friend on the other side of the street. She waves to her friend, who glances her way and then just keeps on walking in the opposite direction. If the woman thinks, "Hmm, she must not have recognized me," she'll probably just go about her business without feeling differently than she did before seeing her friend. But if she thinks, "Wow, what did I do to *her* to make her snub me like that?" she'll end up feeling hurt and resentful and may waste the rest of her day brooding about the perceived rejection. If the woman has SAD, such emotional consequences will only fuel the cycle of negativity that we call depression.

When you're in the midst of SAD symptoms, you can have a lot of negative thoughts about yourself and your circumstances:

"I'm so useless."

"No one should have to be around me."

"I don't like being around other people."

"I'll never get out of this cycle of feeling horrible every winter."

"My family and friends are nice to me only because they feel sorry for me."

"I should be able to rise above this."

You also may be more inclined to misinterpret, exaggerate, or be offended by mundane daily hassles because active depression symptoms lower your resilience and increase your vulnerability. You might feel like your boss is asking too much of you, your children don't appreciate you . . . like little errors are a sign that your character is seriously flawed, that no one loves you. The resentment, hurt, shame, and loneliness that result also feed your SAD symptoms.

Knowing how your own thoughts exacerbate your SAD symptoms gives you an incredibly effective tool for alleviating pain. When you know what thoughts are sending your mood into a nosedive, you can challenge them and, if they're illogi-cal, irrational, or unrealistic, or just plain *wrong,* you can replace them with more realistic, less negative thoughts. With practice the result should be that your mood is either maintained or improved.

⚠ *Unchallenged ANTs Can Become Self-Fulfilling Prophecies*

Negative thoughts like "I'm so useless" and "I'll never get out of this cycle . . . " have a way of coming to fruition when they're allowed to rule your mind unchallenged. A belief that you are useless will make you feel timid, nervous, and depressed, which will make it difficult to take actions that would prove your competence and will leave you paralyzed: prophecy fulfilled.

There are entire self-help books available to help you use CBT methods to change ANTs, and some are listed in the Resources. Or if you think that ANTs might be a major problem for you, you might want to consult a therapist with expertise in CBT. Professional help might be the right route for you if:

- The idea of pursuing a self-help CBT program feels exhausting and overwhelming.

- You're not sure CBT is right for you and want to find out more about other therapies that could help.

How to Choose a Therapist

A therapist you choose to work with should have expertise and experience in CBT (or any other therapeutic method you want to explore). To find a qualified therapist:

- Ask your physician for a referral.

- Ask someone you know who has received therapy for depression or, ideally, specifically for SAD.

- Use the service on the website for the Beck Institute for Cognitive Behavior Therapy or the Academy of Cognitive Therapy (see Resources).

Your therapist should also be responsive, communicative, and a good fit for you. The therapist should:

- Listen attentively and understand what you're saying intellectually and emotionally.

- Be empathic.

- Be thorough in exploring your problem.

- Be open to all treatments proven effective for SAD.

- Have some useful insights or suggestions.

If you're considering trying antidepressants, you might want to seek out a psychiatrist who can not only prescribe but also offer CBT.

- You do better when you're accountable to someone else for completing homework.

- You've tried self-help CBT and end up being stopped by a lot of questions in the middle of the work.

Treat   There are a few different ways you can identify automatic negative thoughts that are worsening your symptoms:

1. Ask yourself whenever you feel your mood descending, "What was I just thinking?" Jot down the thoughts if you like and then see whether a pattern emerges.

2. If you're already using the Daily Mood Log, take a look at what you recorded over a recent month. Look at your low mood ratings and what stressful or exciting events were associated with the dip in mood, and try to reconstruct your thoughts at the time. (Memory isn't flawless, but when an event has been disturbing enough to lower our mood, the same negative thought that arose at the time often pops back up in the mind.) Again, see if you can identify any patterns.

3. Spend a week or so filling out the Thought Log on the facing page to see what types of negative thoughts keep leading to downturns in mood. If you find this process helpful and easy, keep filling it out in the coming weeks.

What Were You Thinking?

All of us have our own brand of negative thinking. Some of us are prone to think in all-or-nothing, black-or-white terms, with no grays. Others operate on a list of inviolable rules about how things "should" be. Psychologists have used lists of 10 or 15 of what are commonly called *cognitive distortions,* or *thinking errors,* to characterize these patterns for more than 30 years. When you can recognize these distortions in your own thinking, you can challenge them. (Mindfulness can also help you accept things as they are, which is why MBCT—see Chapter 12—is so effective.)

Prevent   Following are some common cognitive distortions. After reading about what makes them unrealistic or erroneous, see if your own negative beliefs identified above fit any of these definitions. Think about whether you have often responded in these ways in the past.

Thought Log

At the end of each day, review your day and recall, as well as you can, any events that bothered you. Then write down the thought you reacted with and any change in mood.

Day	Event	Thought(s)	Emotion/mood
Sunday			
Monday			
Tuesday			
Wednesday			
Thursday			
Friday			
Saturday			

Black-or-White Thinking

Most things in life can't be conceptualized as all or nothing, yet some of us try to fit everything into these two extremes. This is the pattern that can lead you to believe that if you're not perfect, you're a complete failure (the tiniest typo on a report, the most minor constructive criticism can send you into a tailspin of self-doubt and depression).

☐ **Are you sometimes an all-or-nothing thinker? Give an example:**

☐ _____

Overgeneralizing

One event guarantees a string of the same. This is the distortion that might lead you to predict, "I'll feel as bad as I did today for every single day this winter."

☐ **Are you sometimes an overgeneralizer? Give an example:**

☐ _____

Filtering Out the Positive

Despite the fact that the day had its ups and downs, the person thinking through a filter sees only the negative: "Not one good thing happened to me today." A variation on this theme is discounting the positive: You recognize it but insist it "doesn't count."

☐ **Do you filter out the positive and focus only on the negative? Give an example:**

☐ _____

Jumping to Conclusions

We're all mind readers or fortune-tellers sometimes. But if you think this way often, you might constantly interpret others' behavior as a sign that they don't like you, can't stand to be around you, feel sorry for you, and so on, despite the fact that you can't read their minds. Or you might say, like the person quoted above, "I'll never get out of this cycle of feeling horrible every winter."

☐ **Are you a mind reader or a fortune-teller? Give an example:**

☐ _____

Catastrophizing

The worst is always going to happen, according to this kind of thinking. You might maximize an impact ("I made such a huge mistake on that report that I'm bound to be fired!") or minimize one ("No one will care that I got a perfect score on the SAT—I still won't get into a good college").

☐ **Do you tend to catastrophize? Give an example:**

☐ _____

Personalization

You're to blame for things you can't possibly control. If you can't seem to give up the idea that having SAD is all your fault, you're personalizing.

☐ **Do you engage in personalization? Give an example:**

☐ _____

Emotional Reasoning

Your emotions are facts. If you dread that spring will never come, you believe you really won't feel better once May arrives (despite the fact that you've felt better in May every year).

☐ **Do you engage in emotional reasoning? Give an example:**

☐ _____

Shoulds

You impose very high standards on yourself and on others. As a result, you end up feeling guilty when you don't live up to them ("I should have been able to pull myself together to go to Marnie's birthday party since she's my best friend") or resentful when others don't ("Tim made it impossible for me to get that report done—he should have known I'd need extra time").

☐ **Do you think in *shoulds*? Give an example:**

☐ _____

Labeling

You attach names (often inaccurate ones) to characterize yourself or someone else rather than just objectively describing what you or the other person did ("I'm a lazy bum" instead of "I couldn't find the energy to do those chores this morning").

☐ **Do you use labeling? Give an example:**

☐ _____

*   *   *

Accurately identifying the cognitive distortions you tend to use isn't easy, but being aware that we all use them can prevent some ANTs from bugging you. Practice as much as you feel able by continuing to log your own negative thoughts. This is also an area where a CBT therapist can help tremendously.

Challenging Automatic Thoughts

Fortunately, negative automatic thoughts can be challenged and replaced with ones that will help, not hinder, your abilities to cope with SAD. Again, this takes a bit of concerted effort, but you can tackle this type of CBT "homework" just a few minutes at a time. Try to do this once a day.

1. If you've been using a thought log, take a quick look at the ones you've filled in and pick one incident where your mood was most severely affected.

2. Thinking back to that event, rate on a scale of 1–10 how strongly you believed the thought that followed the event. If you like, jot that number next to the thought.

3. Now challenge the thought, as if you were cross-examining your own mind.

- What evidence do you have that supports the thought?
- What evidence do you have that refutes the thought?
- What's the worst thing that could happen regarding this thought? The best? The most realistic?
- How could you have handled the event to solve the problem created?

What Advice Would You Give to Someone You Care About?

It can be tough to remove yourself enough from the situation and the thought process to view the whole quick sequence objectively. Try to take yourself out of the equation and pretend a friend or relative has come to you to ask you how to solve the problem that the event created. What advice would you offer?

Treat

Replacing Automatic Thoughts

Now here's the important part:

1. Come up with a new, rational thought to replace the old negative thought, based on the "cross-examination" you just did.

2. Assign it a rating of 1–10 for how strongly you believe it. (You can use the form on page 238 to add your new thought and its rating, plus the impact on your mood, if you like.)

3. Look back at your old automatic thought and rate it again now that you have a rational thought as an alternative. Is it lower?

4. See how your new, rational thought affects your emotions and mood. Do you feel less depressed? Has the new thought generated any positive emotions?

If you don't believe pretty strongly in your new rational thought, it's not a good alternative! If your rating for the new thought is low, try the challenging process again to generate a new thought. Keep trying until you come up with one until you rate it highly and it changes your emotional response in a positive direction.

Let's look at an example using the thought "I'll never get out of this cycle of feeling horrible every winter." Dan woke up Tuesday morning feeling like he could

Thought Log with New, Rational Thoughts

Day	Event	Thought(s)	Emotion/mood	Rational thought	Emotion/mood
Sunday					
Monday					
Tuesday					
Wednesday					
Thursday					
Friday					
Saturday					

barely get up. Before he did wrench himself out of bed, lots of gloomy predictions ran through his mind, all centering on the idea that his SAD would never get better and he'd have to anticipate feeling like this every winter. That made him feel hopeless and even more depressed than when he awoke. This thought felt extremely believable to him. Here's how he filled out his Thought Log:

Day	Event	Thought(s)	Emotion/mood
Tuesday	Woke up feeling terrible after having a good day yesterday	I'll never get out of this cycle of feeling horrible every winter. 9	Hopeless, really depressed

In challenging the thought, Dan looked at the evidence in favor of the thought and came up with the fact that he still had SAD every winter, even though he had been using light therapy and taken steps to reduce his stress and the fact that he still had lots of mornings like this one. To refute the thought, he came up with the fact that he had felt much better yesterday and that if he really looked back at the last winter and this one, he had been able to do things he had not done in earlier winters, like go out with friends at least once most weekends and avoid gaining weight thanks to avoiding carbs and committing to exercise.

If the worst proved true, he realized he'd make a bigger commitment to learning how to cope, mainly by planning during the spring and summer. If the best happened, he'd be rid of SAD forever and live a long and happy life year-round. Realistically, based on the evidence, he figured he might always have to plan for SAD but could keep working at coping and prevention methods, and eventually it might not hold him back so much during winter.

To figure out what he could have done to prevent these thoughts from taking hold if he woke up depressed and groggy, he brainstormed, with the help of his sister, who was his biggest supporter and confidante, and came up with this list.

> *Remember, CBT and all treatments for SAD work better in the light than in the dark!*

- Push myself out of bed the minute a thought like this one enters my head so it doesn't get worse.

- Get a dawn simulator or put a couple of lamps with high-wattage bulbs on a timer so that I get some beneficial effects of light before fully waking up.

- Consider learning mindfulness, which might help me learn to stay in the moment instead of jumping to conclusions about what my current mood means for the future.

- Review the cognitive distortions: "My automatic negative thought seems to have some fortune-telling in it too." "I need to become more aware of when these thinking patterns are taking over."

Dan considered his new thought in this light and actually felt a little hopeful. He said it felt like a weight had been lifted from his shoulders and he could picture being able to get through the day. Here's what his new thought log looked like:

Day	Event	Thought(s)	Emotion/ mood	Rational thought	Emotion/ mood
Tuesday	Woke up feeling terrible after having a good day yesterday	I'll never get out of this cycle of feeling horrible every winter. 3	Hopeless, really depressed	If I get going, I can shrug off this sense of doom and start using my coping methods. 8	Groggy but with a glimmer of hope; lighter than when I opened my eyes

You (and Dan) can now continue the process, challenging other highly rated automatic thoughts and replacing them with new thoughts that you can adopt with conviction. It's hard to strike a balance between not doing enough and making CBT too much work, because it does involve some effort. This is where a coach (a therapist) can help—by sharing the workload with you. We hope you will find, once you try some of the exercises in this chapter, that the benefits make the effort worthwhile and you'll keep it up. Otherwise, maybe you can adopt some of the ideas, work on some over the summer, or consider working with a therapist, which will at least provide you with ongoing support and coaching.

There's one last step in CBT that you can take if and when you're reading. Ask yourself: What's at the root of all these negative thoughts? Where do they come from?

HELPFUL BELIEFS

Negative thoughts don't just pop up out of nowhere. Sure, they are self-perpetuating, so they might just seem like habits of thinking, and they are. But just as low mood is fed by ANTs, ANTs are fueled by negative core beliefs. We all have deeply held beliefs about ourselves, about others, and about the world. These beliefs often involve *should*s and often magically transform themselves into rules that we live by—and expect others to live by, whether or not these are their rules too.

Treat If you feel like looking further at the thoughts that lower your mood and contribute to SAD symptoms, try to identify core beliefs that are the underlying themes behind ANTs. These beliefs hum along in the background like a computer program that governs pop-ups or a word-processing function that dictates how the words you type appear in your document. If you feel deeply that you're not good enough, you might take unjust criticisms to heart or avoid asking for what you need to feel better. If you believe people don't like you, you might avoid social interactions that could give your mood a boost. If you believe that things will always be too difficult, you might pass on opportunities that could improve your symptoms and your life. Core beliefs can be challenged in the same way as negative thoughts. You can create a worksheet similar to the Thought Log with New, Rational Thoughts, or you can just mull this over. Be aware, however, that CBT is known to be most effective when you write everything down.

As an example, let's continue with Dan's negative thought: "I'll never get out of this cycle of feeling horrible every winter." When he looked at his Thought Logs, Dan discovered that his ANTs often reflected a view of the universe as a somewhat hostile, unforgiving place and of himself as helpless to change that. Dan started out challenging the belief "I can't do anything to keep the world from beating me down." He wrote down evidence that supported the belief—including the fact that he had SAD to begin with and that he had been unable to get rid of it to the extent he wanted to. Evidence against the belief that he wrote down included the fact that he had gotten a job he liked after the economic downturn of the 2000s forced his former employer to lay him off and that when he was injured in an accident caused by a drunk driver he became active in the organization MADD. Then he wrote down a new belief: "There's a lot in the world that I can't change, but I can pick a few things that really matter to me and make some difference."

Core beliefs are stubborn, so we have to work hard to release their grip on us. When he started out, Dan was completely (95%) convinced of his core belief. After reviewing the evidence for and against it, he shifted to being 50% convinced of his new core belief. To shift more toward his new belief, he revisited his log every week, considered whether he had any new evidence for or against his original belief, and again rated his old and new beliefs. Gradually his conviction shifted in the direction of the new belief, which also gradually motivated him to keep trying to work on new SAD coping methods.

WHAT HAVE YOU LEARNED ABOUT REPLACING NEGATIVE THOUGHTS AND BELIEFS WITH HELPFUL ONES?

Sometimes writing down what you gained (or where your expectations weren't met) helps gel your thoughts and stimulate new ideas. If you think it might help you plan for next year, jot down a few thoughts about any particular automatic negative thoughts (ANTs) that have played a big role in permitting SAD symptoms to keep you down, how you'll keep using the tools in this chapter to replace negative thoughts and beliefs, and how these measures have helped you make inroads into SAD:

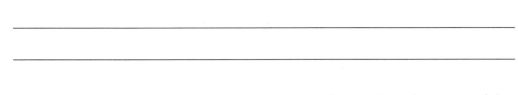

Adding this information to your action plan in Chapter 6 can keep it useful as an up-to-date reference.

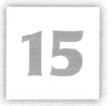

15

Medication for SAD

WHAT DO YOU HOPE TO GET OUT OF ANTIDEPRESSANT MEDICATION?

☐ I can't tolerate light therapy and need something else with proven effectiveness for SAD.

☐ Light therapy has reduced my symptoms somewhat, stress management has helped me cope, but I really need more to be able to get through winter days reasonably well.

☐ I don't have the energy to try psychotherapy, and I've struggled through more miserable winters than I can count. I need to do something that doesn't require even more effort and might help me quickly.

☐ I'm looking for prevention. Once my symptoms get into full swing, I seem to lose all my abilities to help myself.

★ KEY POINTS

Antidepressant medication is an effective treatment that should be considered when other remedies are not enough to help you take your life back from SAD.

*　　*　　*

Antidepressant medications have been a godsend to millions of individuals suffering from all kinds of depression, including SAD. They are particularly useful when symptoms are severe and rob the person of the energy and focus necessary to undertake psychotherapy such as CBT. The same principle applies to those with SAD. Because, however, many people with SAD get at least some improvement quickly from light therapy, antidepressants for SAD may not be the best treatment to try first, but second or third. Most people with SAD can get significant benefit from a combination of light therapy, an antidepressant medication, and various other strategies described in earlier chapters. Many people, however, get sufficient improvement from light therapy, stress management techniques, and lifestyle modifications, and medication may be unnecessary. However, even if other methods will do the job, adding medication may still make sense because of how easy it is to take pills and how effective they often are.

↗ FAST FACTS

- Dozens of studies have shown positive effects of antidepressant medications in people with SAD (even though the number of subjects in most of these studies has been small).

- Antidepressants are thought to work by correcting an imbalance in serotonin, dopamine, and/or norepinephrine in the brain.

- If one antidepressant doesn't help you, another might, depending on your unique brain chemistry.

- Antidepressants can help whether they are started before or after SAD symptoms appear.

HOW TO DECIDE WHETHER TO TRY ANTIDEPRESSANTS

The decision to take (or not take) medication is always yours, but it will be a well-informed choice if made in collaboration with a practitioner who knows you well and thoroughly understands the workings of antidepressants. In this chapter you'll find some factors to consider and questions to ask that will help you weigh the pros and cons, as well as tools to use during a trial of medication that will enable you to collaborate effectively in your own care. Finding a professional who knows how to use antidepressants can be relatively easy, which is good news if you're interested in pursuing medication. It's often more difficult, however, to find someone who knows all the different treatments and how to blend them.

What type of physician will be most helpful to you?

- A doctor you trust: Being able to work together and communicate clearly is a must if you hope to get optimal advice and support.

- A psychiatrist with experience in treating SAD: This would be the ideal because a doctor with these qualifications will have the greatest knowledge to offer you, but it may not be feasible if no such professional is easily accessible to you.

- Your primary care physician: If your physician is amenable and has prescribed antidepressants for other types of depression, he or she might be able to prescribe and monitor your medication. If the doctor expresses any hesitation, however, ask for a referral.

- A physician assistant or nurse practitioner: In most states these professionals are permitted to prescribe medication. If your health care providers work in a group setting that includes PAs or NPs, you may already be regularly consulting one of these practitioners and can work with him or her on SAD medication as well.

Here are some questions you can ask a practitioner:

- Have you treated SAD before, and if so, how often with medication?

- How successful do you think these treatments have been?

- What do you think the advantages of medication are for SAD?

- How do you determine who is a good candidate for an antidepressant?

- What do I need to know about a medication trial for SAD?

- How long will it take me to feel any benefits?

- What kinds of side effects should I expect?

- What will you advise if I try an antidepressant and it doesn't work or I have intolerable side effects?

- Are there any additional adverse effects of taking these medications long term?

- Will I need to change anything else that I do while taking one of these medications?

Debunking Myths about Medications for SAD

- "I'll get hooked": Antidepressant medications are not addictive.

- "I'll turn into someone else": These medications generally do not change one's personality or alter thinking and behavior in any radical way. They are designed to ease the symptoms of depression by acting on neurotransmitters involved in depression.

- "Taking drugs is the easy way out and would be a sign of character weakness": A well-considered decision to try medication is not an easy way out; it's a smart way to help yourself. This type of attitude is often a product of negative core beliefs that can stand in the way of your getting the help you need (see Chapter 14).

- "If I start taking these pills, I'll be dependent on them for the rest of my life": If you have severe SAD, there is a chance that you will want to take an antidepressant for the rest of your life, or certainly for as long as your symptoms recur without medication. (Many people who need medicine for SAD during the winter are, however, able to discontinue them in spring.) Diabetics depend on insulin, those with hypertension often depend on medications to lower blood pressure, and people with vision problems may depend (barring corrective surgery) on eyeglasses. Does that mean they should deny themselves what they need? Or be ashamed of needing it? Again, this kind of concern may be based on a negative core belief that is only standing in your way of being treated for something that isn't your fault (see Chapter 14).

You are a potential candidate for antidepressant medication if:

- ☑ **Your symptoms are moderate to severe.**

- ☑ **Your overall health is relatively good.**

- ☑ **Light therapy and other measures have proven or seem likely to be insufficient.**

Downsides of antidepressants include:

☑ **Side effects, which are a possibility with all medications.**

☑ **Cost (for both the medicine itself and doctor's appointments).**

HOW ANTIDEPRESSANT MEDICATIONS WORK

Everything controlled by the brain, including regulation of mood, happens when neurons communicate with each other. Spurred by electrical signals in the neurons, chemical messengers called *neurotransmitters* are released into the spaces between two neurons, known as *synapses,* and carry commands from the transmitter neuron to the receptor neuron. Once they have delivered their message ("Be calm!" or "Feel euphoric!"), these neurotransmitters return to the transmitting neuron and are broken down.

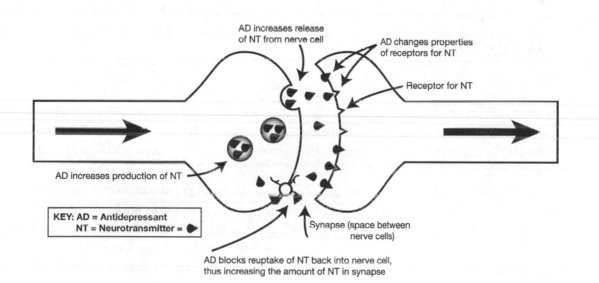

Reprinted with permission from *Breaking Free from Depression: Pathways to Wellness* by Jesse H. Wright and Laura W. McCray (Guilford Press, 2012). Copyright 2012 by The Guilford Press.

Depression is thought to be the result of abnormal actions between neurons by certain neurotransmitters. Therefore most antidepressants, especially the more recently developed ones, are designed to prevent reuptake of certain neurotransmitters that control mood (the return of the neurotransmitter to the transmitting neuron). With more of that neurotransmitter sending its message to the receiving neuron, mood or whatever else is controlled by that neurochemical may be improved.

Three neurotransmitters in particular are instrumental in depression:

Serotonin: Serotonin could be viewed as the serenity chemical. With appropriate levels of serotonin doing their job, you can remain calm, your mood is high, and you aren't too inclined to lose your temper or become agitated.

Dopamine: Dopamine is the pleasure chemical. It also governs the mechanisms for reward, motivation, and attention.

Norepinephrine: Norepinephrine is the energy chemical. With enough of it operating, you feel vital and alert.

It's not too hard to see that, with too little of any of these neurotransmitters doing its job, you'd have some of the symptoms of depression. As noted in Chapter 3, we have evidence that serotonin might be involved in several aspects of SAD (even carb cravings!). Yet the most compelling evidence of effectiveness in SAD is for a medication that affects dopamine and norepinephrine (see the information that follows).

🧪 SCIENCE

Wellbutrin: First Choice for SAD?

In a set of studies I did with GlaxoSmithKline, more than 1,000 people were given the extended-release form of Wellbutrin (bupropion) in the fall, before the onset of their SAD symptoms, to see whether this antidepressant prevented SAD symptoms from starting in winter. This treatment reduced the risk of an episode during winter by almost 50%, and subsequently Wellbutrin XL was approved by the U.S. Food and Drug Administration (FDA) for preventing episodes in those with severe SAD.

Wellbutrin also is less likely to cause the sexual dysfunction, lethargy, and weight gain that are common side effects of the selective serotonin reuptake inhibitors (SSRIs). In fact, Wellbutrin is often energizing and actually causes weight loss, a potential benefit for anyone with SAD-related carb cravings. Caution: Wellbutrin should not be taken by people with a history of seizure disorders.

🧰 TOOLS

Tools You Can Use: An Up-to-Date List of Your Medications

Before your doctor prescribes an antidepressant, your full medical history will be taken, including a list of all the medications you are currently taking. It's a good idea to keep this list updated so that you have it available at all times. Feel free to make extra copies or download the form from *www.guilford.com/rosenthal3-forms*.

My Medications (Prescription and OTC Drugs and Supplements)

Medication: _____ Dosage: _____

taken _____ a day at _____ (times)

Medication: _____ Dosage: _____

taken _____ a day at _____ (times)

Medication: _____ Dosage: _____

taken _____ a day at _____ (times)

Medication: _____ Dosage: _____

taken _____ a day at _____ (times)

Medication: _____ Dosage: _____

taken _____ a day at _____ (times)

Medication: _____ Dosage: _____

taken _____ a day at _____ (times)

Medication: _____ Dosage: _____

taken _____ a day at _____ (times)

Medication: _____ Dosage: _____

taken _____ a day at _____ (times)

Medication: _____ Dosage: _____

taken _____ a day at _____ (times)

Medication: _____ Dosage: _____

taken _____ a day at _____ (times)

Medication: _____ Dosage: _____

taken _____ a day at _____ (times)

New medications should not be prescribed for you without considering possible drug interactions. This list should always include over-the-counter medications, as well as supplements.

HOW A MEDICATION TRIAL WORKS

Antidepressants may take several weeks to exert their full beneficial effect, and sometimes side effects that are troublesome at first level out after a couple of weeks. Generally you should expect a medication trial of one drug to last for 3 weeks *after* the best dose is reached. If your SAD is severe, your doctor may start you at a relatively higher dose right away so that you don't waste a lot of time gradually upping the dose until the best benefits are gained. Otherwise, your doctor will likely start you on the lowest dosage that has been seen to be effective for your specific condition and increase as needed. This means that it could take a couple months to reach the best medication and dosage for you.

If after a series of trials you haven't found one medication that works for you, you may need to take more than one medication at a time. While this happens in a minority of cases, it's not uncommon.

You will be asked to keep track of your symptoms and any side effects, as well as other concerns that arise while you are trying out the prescribed medication(s). A Medication Log you can use for this purpose appears on page 252, or your doctor may provide one. You can certainly keep track more informally, but it's wise to record your experience somewhere (your smartphone may be a good option since you're likely to have it with you all day) because reports about the last few weeks are unlikely to be very reliable or specific when pieced together from memory.

⚠ **Call your doctor before your next appointment if you suffer any severe side effects. Most doctors will discuss the most common side effects with you when proposing a trial of a particular medication, but it's wise to have information on hand about rarer, severe side effects in case one should occur. If your pharmacy is not in the habit of providing the full package insert for a medication, ask for it so that you have it on hand.**

Doctors ask about your current medications before prescribing anything, but if another physician prescribes a new medication for you, be aware that it might interact negatively with your antidepressant, and call your prescribers if you notice a new side effect.

Obviously, caution should be taken to follow the precise instructions on all prescription medications.

TOOLS

Tools You Can Use: Medication Log

You can use the medication log on page 252 both during medication trials and after you and your doctor have decided on a particular medication regimen. (Feel free to make extra copies or download the form from *www.guilford.com/rosenthal3-forms*.) Even once the trial is finished, your reaction to a medication may change over time, especially considering that changes in the brain do occur as the seasons progress in those with SAD. Never hesitate to contact your doctor if your medication no longer seems to be helping or new side effects appear. For instance, some people start to have undesirable side effects, such as overstimulation, when spring is arriving, which is often a signal to start tapering off the medication, under your doctor's supervision.

⚠ *Don't Discontinue an Antidepressant Abruptly!*

You may need to take an antidepressant only during fall and winter, but this is something you should talk to your doctor about ahead of time to come up with a course of action for discontinuing the medication. Suddenly going off an antidepressant can not only bring on depression—although this is often not the case if you are emerging from your SAD season—but also might cause weird dreams, pins and needles, mood swings and irritability, dizziness, and other unpleasant feelings. Your doctor will probably want you to contact him if you begin to feel that you are getting overstimulated or notice other signs that may mean you're no longer depressed enough to need the medication, and then will give you a plan for tapering the medication so that you don't feel any untoward effects.

SPECIFIC MEDICATIONS FOR SAD

The medications in the table on page 253 are listed in the order in which I usually prescribe them for patients, based on effectiveness and side effects. The table shows which neurotransmitters are targeted and sums up advantages and side effects. Here are additional important details about each group of antidepressants. Ask your doctor for more information. Also see the Resources for websites on depression and its treatments and for news on advances in medications for depression in general and SAD in particular.

Medication Log

Date/time	Medication/dosage	Effects on SAD	Side effects	Comments

Brief Overview of Antidepressants

Brand (generic) name	Neurotransmitters affected	Potential advantages	Potential disadvantages
Wellbutrin (bupropion)	DA +++ NE ++	Less likely to cause sexual difficulties and weight gain. Can prevent depression if started early in season.	Not as good for anxiety; may increase risk of seizures in vulnerable individuals.
Selective serotonin reuptake inhibitors (SSRIs)			
Prozac (fluoxetine)	SE +++	All are effective. Approved for some anxiety disorders as well as depression.	Side effects: Problems with sexual functioning, lethargy, weight gain.
Zoloft (sertraline)	SE +++		
Paxil (paroxetine)	SE +++		
Celexa (citalopram)	SE +++		
Luvox (fluvoxamine)	SE +++		
Viibryd (vilazodone)	SE +++		
Serotonin and norepinephrine reuptake inhibitors (SNRIs)			
Effexor (venlafaxine)	SE ++ NE ++	Approved for treatment of some anxiety disorders as well as depression.	Can cause increased blood pressure and some SSRI-type side effects.
Cymbalta (duloxetine)	SE + NE +++	May be helpful when there is pain as well as depression.	Can cause nausea, dry mouth, drowsiness, constipation, and insomnia.
Savella (milnacipran)*	SE + NE +++		

Note. Reprinted with permission from *Winter Blues: Everything You Need to Beat Seasonal Affective Disorder* (4th ed.) by Norman E. Rosenthal (Guilford Press, 2013). Copyright 2013 by Norman E. Rosenthal. SE = serotonin; NE = norepinephrine; DA = dopamine; + = slight; ++ = moderate; +++ = marked.

*At the time of printing this medication was approved for fibromyalgia but not depression in the United States; elsewhere it is approved for both.

$ = brand name only available (still under patent)

¢ = available as a generic

Wellbutrin (bupropion)

★ KEY POINTS

Particularly helpful if SAD makes you very sluggish and lethargic or if you already tend to gain weight in winter.

Forms: immediate (IR), sustained (SR), and extended release (XL). All ¢.

Common side effects: dry mouth, nausea, constipation, flatulence, weight loss.

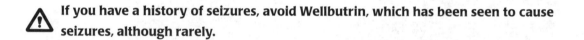 **If you have a history of seizures, avoid Wellbutrin, which has been seen to cause seizures, although rarely.**

Selective Serotonin Reuptake Inhibitors

★ KEY POINTS

Particularly helpful if anxiety is a big part of your SAD.

Brand and chemical names: Prozac (fluoxetine), ¢; Zoloft (sertraline), ¢; Paxil (paroxetine), ¢; Luvox (fluvoxamine), $; Celexa (citalopram), ¢; Lexapro (escitalopram), ¢.

Side effects: sexual dysfunction (decreased desire, problems with arousal and achieving orgasm), flat emotions, fatigue, weight gain.

Serotonin and Norepinepherine Reuptake Inhibitors

★ KEY POINTS

Particularly helpful if pain is part of your SAD.

⚠️ **Those who drink excessively may suffer liver damage from Cymbalta and should avoid it.**

Brand and chemical names: Effexor (venlafaxine), ¢; Cymbalta (duloxetine), $.

Forms: immediate (IR) and extended release (XR) for Effexor; immediate release (IR) only for Cymbalta

Side effects: Cymbalta—nausea, constipation, dry mouth, drowsiness, insomnia, high blood pressure; Effexor—edginess, sedation, high blood pressure, sleep disruption, sexual dysfunction

Tricyclic Antidepressants

★ KEY POINTS

Useful mainly if, for whatever reason, Wellbutrin, SSRIs, and SNRIs cannot help with your SAD.

⚠️ **TCAs can be fatal in overdose and must be used with extreme care.**

Tricyclic antidepressants were the only choice before the SSRIs and their kin came along. I hardly ever prescribe them for SAD because the newer drugs are effective without the problematic side effects or overdose danger.

Brand and chemical names: Norpramin (desipramine), ¢, Tofranil (imipramine), ¢, Pamelor (nortriptyline) ¢, Elavil (amitriptyline), ¢.

⚗ SCIENCE

Stay Tuned . . .

Watch for news about studies of new antidepressants in the treatment of SAD. Three newer drugs that have come on the market are Viibryd (vilazodone), which operates on serotonin and is approved in the United States as an antidepressant; Savella (milnacipran), which operates on both serotonin and norepinephrine but is approved in the United States only for fibromyalgia, and Valdoxan (agomelatine), which operates on melatonin and serotonin receptors but has not yet been approved in the United States. The Internet (see the Resources for reliable sources of information) is the most up-to-date source of information on recent research and FDA approval.

WHAT HAVE YOU LEARNED ABOUT ANTIDEPRESSANT MEDICATIONS FOR SAD?

Sometimes writing down what you gained (or where your expectations weren't met) helps gel your thoughts and stimulate new ideas. If you think it might help you plan for next year, jot down a few thoughts about how medication might help you (if at all), how you might combine it with other treatments and strategies, and how you can work with your doctor.

_____

_____

_____

Adding this information to your action plan in Chapter 6 can keep it useful as an up-to-date reference.

What I Would Like You to Know about SAD

Seasonal affective disorder (SAD) is a form of depression that affects women, men, and children around the world, particularly in the Northern Hemisphere. People with SAD react to the change of seasons, and particularly to short and dark days, with low mood, irritability, sluggishness, lack of energy, difficulty concentrating, and changes in sleep and eating patterns. About 5% of adults in the northern regions of Europe and North America qualify for a diagnosis of SAD, and 14% more have a milder version of the problem, often referred to informally as "the winter blues." SAD is four times more common in women than in men. Although it is biologically based, it is aggravated by stress as well as darkness. It is sometimes inherited, and in women it is most frequently a problem during the reproductive years, although children and older adults also can have SAD symptoms.

Many people have SAD for years before receiving help, believing the problem is a sign of personal weakness or failure instead of the legitimate illness that it is. Unfortunately, lack of treatment can cause people to:

- Lose productive work days and effectiveness in all areas

- Withdraw from others

- Sleep too much

- Eat too much and gain weight

- Become couch potatoes due to lack of energy

- Lose interest in sex

- Become despondent and, in rare cases, even have suicidal thoughts

Fortunately, symptoms can be lessened, reversed, and sometimes even prevented with proven treatments:

More Light

This is the most effective and most important treatment for most people with SAD. Exposure to light can be increased through:

- Light therapy using a light box for 20–45 minutes once or twice a day
- Adding light to the environment, through clean windows, extra artificial lighting at home and at work, and even bright decor
- Vacations in sunny locales to break up the winter

Stress Management

Symptoms can be alleviated with planning to:

- Cut back on obligations and manage time well during the season of risk
- Add pleasant activities to daily life
- Pursue exercise (especially outdoors in sunlight)
- Manage diet to avoid weight gain caused by carbohydrate cravings
- Practice meditation and relaxation
- Get help and support from friends, family, and coworkers

Medication

Antidepressant medications can help people who don't get sufficient improvement from light therapy and stress management.

With trial and error and planning, most people with SAD can arrive at a combination of treatments and remedies that will allow them to lead satisfying lives throughout the year. You can help them maintain their role in your life and stay healthy and productive just by understanding why the person needs to adjust his or her routine and responsibilities during the season of active symptoms and accommodating those needs in whatever ways are possible and reasonable.

Resources

www.normanrosenthal.com

On my personal website I provide regular updates on SAD and its treatment, as well as other aspects of my work. My blog offers help and support on a number of issues of interest to people with SAD and others.

Center for Environmental Therapeutics
www.cet.org

The CET website provides a broad variety of resources for individuals and professionals on light therapy, dawn simulation, and negative air ionization. In addition to information about therapeutic devices, you'll find online assessments for SAD, circadian rhythm types, and depression overall and information through various media.

National Institute of Mental Health
www.nimh.nih.gov

The NIMH website includes a broad range of up-to-date information on depression (and other disorders): ongoing research and research findings, publications, support, psychoeducation, and more.

National Alliance on Mental Illness
www.nami.org

NAMI is a large grassroots mental health organization dedicated to advocacy and awareness. A wealth of resources is offered on its website and through its state and local affiliates.

Depression and Bipolar Support Alliance
www.dbsalliance.org

DBSA provides help, support, and information for people with mood disorders, including news, treatment information, peer support, and an extensive library, including helpful podcasts.

Mood Disorders Society of Canada
www.mooddisorderscanada.ca
This organization's website offers support and advocacy for those with mood disorders in Canada, including links to support groups and national and provincial organizations.

Depression Alliance
www.depressionalliance.org
Depression Alliance provides extensive information on depression and multiple links to support groups all over the United Kingdom.

SAD SUPPORT GROUPS

Seasonal Affective Disorder Association
www.sada.org.uk
SADA, the oldest support group for SAD, has been in operation for decades, during which it has served hundreds of thousands of people. It is an exemplary nonprofit organization that is well worth looking into, especially if you live in the United Kingdom. In many instances a support group can be established through the persistence of a single individual, who then inspires many others to follow her or his example. In the case of SADA, Jennifer Eastwood was the founding member, although dozens of dedicated volunteers have kept the organization going since its inception.

SAD in Sweden
www.sadinsweden.com
More recently, Esther O'Hara, formerly of the United Kingdom and now living in Sweden, appealed to SADA to help her start a Swedish support group. Contact her at Esther O'Hara, Von Döbelns Väg 56, 461 58 Trollhättan, Sweden; e-mail: *estherohara@ gmail.com.*

SOURCES OF THERAPEUTIC DEVICES AND OTHER EQUIPMENT

The following manufacturers have long track records for quality control, reliability, and willingness to stand by their products, but there are many other companies and products you can review online with a variety of light fixtures and other devices. Just be sure that any equipment you buy comes with a full money-back guarantee within 30 days if you are not satisfied with the product for any reason. *When you receive your purchase, be sure to record the expiration date for your money-back guarantee in the spot provided in Chapter 7, and file your receipt and warranty in a safe place.*

SunBox Company
19217 Orbit Drive
Gaithersburg, MD 20879
Phone: 301-869-5980
Toll-free: 800-LITE-YOU (548-3968)
www.sunbox.com
e-mail: *info@sunbox.com*
    Besides light boxes, dawn simulators, light visors, light pipes, and negative ion generators can also be obtained from SunBox.

Northern Light Technologies
8971 Henri Bourassa West
St. Laurent PQ, H4S 1P7, Canada
Phone: 514-335-1763
Toll-free: 800-263 0066
Fax: 514-335-7764
www.northernlighttechnologies.com
e-mail: *info@northernlight-tech.com*

Verilux, Inc.
The Healthy Lighting Company
340 Mad River Park
Waitsfield, VT 05673
Phone: 802-496-3101
Toll-free: 800-454-4408
Fax: 802-496-3105
www.verilux.com

Also see the Center for Environmental Therapeutics, listed above.

For skylight alternatives to let extra daylight into your residence through the roof, here are a couple of companies, but be sure to search the Internet for other possibilities (or consult local roofing companies):

The Sun Pipe Company, Inc.
http://sunpipe-original.com

Solatube International, Inc.
2210 Oak Ridge Way
Vista, CA 92081-8341
Toll-free: 888-765-2882
www.solatube.com

SAD, LIGHT THERAPY, AND RELATED TOPICS

Lam, R. W. (1998). *Seasonal Affective Disorder and Beyond: Light Treatment for SAD and Non-SAD Conditions.* Washington, DC: American Psychiatric Press.

Lam, R. W., and Levitt, A. J. (Eds.). (1999). *Clinical Guidelines for the Treatment of Seasonal Affective Disorder.* Washington, DC: American Psychiatric Press.

Oren, D. A., Reich, W., Rosenthal, N. E., and Wehr, T. A. (2006). *How to Beat Jet Lag: A Practical Guide for Air Travelers.* New York: Henry Holt.

Rosenthal, N. (2013). *Winter Blues: Everything You Need to Know to Beat Seasonal Affective Disorder.* 4th edition. New York: Guilford Press. —This comprehensive volume contains detailed information and research findings on all things SAD.

Rosenthal, N. E., and Blehar, M. (1989). *Seasonal Affective Disorders and Phototherapy.* New York: Guilford Press. —This was the first compilation of papers on SAD and light therapy and contains papers about the history of SAD and other aspects of the early thinking on the subject that will be of interest to scholars.

Rosenthal, N. E., Sack, D. A., Gillin, J. C., Lewy, A. J., Goodwin, F. K., Davenport, Y., et al. (1984). Seasonal affective disorder: A description of the syndrome and preliminary findings with light therapy. *Archives of General Psychiatry, 41*(1), 72–80. —This is the original description of SAD and its treatment with light therapy.

Terman, M.,and McMahan, I. (2012). *The Inner Clock: Using Chronobiology to Boost Your Mood, Energy and Sleep Quality.* New York: Avery/Penguin.

Wirz-Justice, A., Benedetti, F., and Terman, M. (2009). *Chronotherapeutics for Affective Disorders.* Basel, Switzerland: Karger.

ADDITIONAL INFORMATION AND HELP FOR SPECIFIC NEEDS

Time Management

Mind Tools
www.mindtools.com

A comprehensive selection of tools for not only time management but also stress management, creativity (brainstorming and problem-solving skills can be extremely helpful in managing SAD), decision making, and more.

Diet

Agatston, A. (2005). *The South Beach Diet: The Delicious, Doctor-Designed, Foolproof Plan for Fast and Healthy Weight Loss.* New York: St. Martin's Griffin.

Agatston, A. (2010). *The South Beach Diet Super Quick Cookbook: 200 Easy Solutions for Everyday Meals.* New York: St. Martin's.
—*www.southbeachdiet.com*

Atkins, R. C. (2002). *Dr. Atkins' New Diet Revolution, Revised Edition.* Lanham, MD: M. Evans & Company.

Atkins, R. C. (2004). *Atkins for Life: The Complete Controlled Carb Program for Permanent Weight Loss and Good Health*. New York: Martin's Griffin.
—*www.atkins.com*

Atkins Health & Medical Information Service. (2004). *The Atkins Shopping Guide: Indispensable Tips and Guidelines for Successfully Stocking Your Low-Carb Kitchen*. New York: Avon.

Bowden, J. (2005). *Living Low-Carb: Controlled Carbohydrate Eating for Long-Term Weight Loss*. New York: Sterling.

Eades, M. R., and Eades, M. D. (1999). *Protein Power: The High-Protein/Low-Carbohydrate Way to Lose Weight, Feel Fit, and Boost Your Health—in Just Weeks!* New York: Bantam.
—*www.proteinpower.com*

Leighton, H., Bethea, M. C., Andrews, S. S., and Balart, L. A. (2001). *Sugar Busters!: Cut Sugar to Trim Fat*. New York: Ballantine.
—*www.sugarbusters.com*

Peeke, P. (2012). *The Hunger Fix: The 3-Stage Detox and Recovery Plan for Overeating and Food Addiction*. Emmaus, PA: Rodale Press.

Sears, B., and Lawren, B. (1995). *Enter The Zone: A Dietary Road Map*. New York: Regan.

Sears, B., and Sears, L. (2004). *Zone Meals in Seconds: 150 Fast and Delicious Recipes for Breakfast, Lunch, and Dinner*. New York: William Morrow.
—*www.zonediet.com*

Willett, W. C. (2005). *Eat, Drink and Be Healthy: The Harvard Medical School Guide to Healthy Eating*. New York: Free Press.

Meditation

Ekirch, A. R. (2005). *At Day's Close: Night in Times Past*. New York: Norton.

Germer, C. K. (2009). *The Mindful Path to Self-Compassion: Freeing Yourself from Destructive Thoughts and Emotions*. New York: Guilford Press.
—*www.mindfulselfcompassion.org* (includes downloads of mindfulness exercises)

Gunaratana, B. H. (2010). *Mindfulness in Plain English*. Somerville, MA: Wisdom Publications.

Hofman, S. G., Sawyer, A. T., Witt, A. A., Oh, D. (2010). The effect of mindfulness-based therapy on anxiety and depression: A meta-analytic review. *Journal of Consulting and Clinical Psychology, 78*(2), 169–183.

Rosenthal, N. E. (2011). *Transcendence: Healing and Transformation through Transcendental Meditation*. New York: Tarcher Penguin.

Shear, J. (Ed.). (2006). *The Experience of Meditation: Experts Introduce the Major Traditions*. St. Paul, MN: Paragon House.

Siegel, R. D. (2010). *The Mindfulness Solution: Everyday Practices for Everyday Problems*. New York: Guilford Press.

Teasdale, J., Segal, Z., and Williams, M. (2014). *The Mindful Way Workbook: An 8-Week Program to Free Yourself from Depression and Emotional Distress*. New York: Guilford Press.

Warren, J. (2007). *The Head Trip: Adventures on the Wheel of Consciousness*. New York: Random House.

Williams, M., Teasdale, J., Segal, Z., and Kabat–Zinn, J. (2007). *The Mindful Way through Depression: Freeing Yourself from Chronic Unhappiness.* New York: Guilford Press.

For more information check out: *www.tm.org* and *www.davidlynchfoundation.org*

Pleasant Activities

www.robertjmeyersphd.com/download/Pleasant%20Activities%20List%20(PAL).pdf
www.raleighpsychology.com/pleasant.htm
www.dodgydigital.com/frank_mcdonald/Depression_files/Pleasantactivities.pdf

Cognitive-Behavioral Therapy

Academy of Cognitive Therapy
www.academyofct.org

Beck Institute for Cognitive Behavior Therapy
www.beckinstitute.org

Burns, D. D. (1999). *Feeling Good: The New Mood Therapy.* New York: Harper.
Rohan, K. J. (2008). *Coping with the Seasons: A Cognitive Behavioral Approach to Seasonal Affective Disorder, Workbook.* New York: Oxford University Press.

Also see Teasdale et al. (2014), listed above.

Positive Psychology

Seligman, M. E. P. (1998). *Learned Optimism* (2nd ed.). New York: Pocket Books.
Seligman, M. E. P., and Csikszentmihalyi, M. (2000). Positive psychology: An introduction. *American Psychologist, 55*(1), 5–14.

Index

About the Authors

Norman E. Rosenthal, MD, is internationally recognized for his pioneering contributions to understanding SAD and using light therapy to treat it. He is Clinical Professor of Psychiatry at Georgetown Medical School, a therapist in private practice, and the author of six other books, including *Winter Blues,* the *New York Times* bestseller *Transcendence,* and *The Gift of Adversity.* Dr. Rosenthal conducted research at the National Institute of Mental Health for over 20 years and is a highly cited researcher.

Christine M. Benton is a freelance writer and editor who lives and works in Chicago.